W0043731

URINARY TRACT INFECTIONS

PRACTICAL CLINICAL MEDICINE

Series Editors J. Fry and G. Sandler

URINARY TRACT INFECTIONS

Edited by D. Brooks

*General Practitioner, Middleton, Manchester
and Associate Advisor in General Practice,
Department of Postgraduate Medical Studies,
University of Manchester*

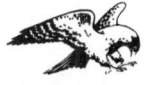 **MTP PRESS LIMITED**
a member of the KLUWER ACADEMIC PUBLISHERS GROUP
LANCASTER / BOSTON / THE HAGUE / DORDRECHT

Published in the UK and Europe by
MTP Press Limited
Falcon House
Lancaster, England

British Library Cataloguing in Publication Data
Urinary tract infections.—(Practical
   clinical medicine).
   1. Urinary organs—Diseases
   I. Brooks, David, *1939–*   II. Series
   616.6   RC900

   ISBN-13: 978-0-85200-695-5   e-ISBN-13: 978-94-010-9932-5
   DOI: 10.1007/978-94-010-9932-5

Published in the USA by
MTP Press
A division of Kluwer Academic Publishers
101 Philip Drive
Norwell, MA 02061, USA

Library of Congress Cataloging in Publication Data
Urinary tract infections.

   (Practical clinical medicine)
   Includes bibliographies and index.
   1. Urinary tract infections. I. Brooks,
David. II. Series. [DNLM: 1. Urinary Tract
Infections. WJ 151 U7621]
RC901.8.U75   1987   616.6   87–4115
ISBN-13: 978-0-85200-695-5

Copyright © 1987 MTP Press Limited
All rights reserved. No part of this publication may be reproduced, stored
in a retrieval system, or transmitted in any form or by any means, electronic,
mechanical, photocopying, recording or otherwise, without prior permission
from the publishers.

Butler & Tanner Limited, Frome and London

Contents

List of Contributors

J. C. Brocklehurst, MD, FRCP,
Consultant Physician,
Withington Hospital,
Manchester;
Professor of Geriatric
Medicine,
University of Manchester

D. Brooks, MD, FRCGP, DObstRCOG,
General Practitioner,
Middleton, Manchester;
Associate Advisor in General
Practice,
Department of Postgraduate
Medical Studies,
University of Manchester

S. L. Choudhury, BSc, MRCP,
Consultant Physician in
Geriatric Medicine,
Chester City Hospital,
Chester

T. C. O'Dowd, MD, MRCGP,
Senior Lecturer in General
Practice,
University of Nottingham,
Queen's Medical Centre,
Nottingham

R. J. Postlethwaite, MBChB,
FRCP, Consultant Paediatric
Nephrologist, Royal
Manchester
Children's Hospital,
Pendlebury and Booth Hall
Hospital, Manchester

P. Smith, MCh, FRCS,
Consultant Urologist,
Bristol Royal Infirmary,
Bristol

Series Editors' Foreword

Backing up the pioneering medical researchers and experi-
menters are the phalanxes and cohorts of practising clinicians
in district general hospitals and in general practice who may
have to implement and apply any breakthroughs and advances
in practical and realistic terms. This they cannot, and should
not, be expected to do without careful consideration and
analysis. It is essential, therefore, to have regular reviews of
the growing points of medicine which are constructively critical
as well as being enthusiastic and which can present the issues
and implications clearly and fairly to clinicians.

The *Practical Clinical Medicine* series is designed to provide
such regular reviews on selected subjects. Each volume is under
the charge of an invited editor who selects his team of 4–6
experts. Each contribution is an authoritative, detailed and
referenced examination of his topic, is clearly presented in an
understandable manner and is practical, relevant and applicable to everyday clinical practice.

The series is intended as a means of communication between
researchers and practising clinicians. It is dedicated to generalists who provide primary health care in general practice and
to generalists providing secondary medical care in district

general hospitals. Both are involved in applying good general practical clinical medicine for their patients, but can only succeed in a climate of constant review and examination.

JOHN FRY
GERALD SANDLER

Preface

This is essentially a book which editor and contributors hope will lead to the better management of general practice patients who present with symptoms of urinary tract infection. The authors all have research and clinical experience in their fields and are very familiar with the problems faced by general practitioners. They have addressed practical questions, as follows.

Chapter One *Concepts, Definitions and their Practical Value – An Overview*

Questions
  (1) What is urinary tract infection?
  (2) What organisms are involved?
  (3) Why don't we all get urinary tract infection?
  (4) How do we know it is there?
  (5) How should the general practitioner approach a diagnosis?

Chapter Two   *Women with Urinary Symptoms*

Questions
  (1) What should our objectives be when we take a history?
  (2) Is there any point in examining the patient?
  (3) If so, what procedures should we carry out and why?
  (4) Do patients with symptoms need to be investigated bac-
      teriologically in general practice? If they do, is it because
      the disease is serious so that reliable information is needed
      about its presence or absence if the right patients are
      to be referred to hospital, or is it because therapeutic
      intervention is a serious matter and reliable information
      is necessary to support it?
  (5) Which drugs should we use and for how long should
      women be treated?
  (6) What do we say to our women patients?
  (7) Is follow-up with or without urine investigation necess-
      ary?
  (8) What are the indications for referral and to what sort of
      specialist should women be referred?
  (9) Is screening necessary/desirable/a waste of resources?

Chapter Three   *Men with Urinary Tract Infection*

Questions
  (1) What should we look for in the history?
  (2) How should we examine the patient?
  (3) Should we obtain a urine specimen? What should we look
      for and how should we interpret the report?
  (4) Is there a drug(s) of choice and for how long should drug
      treatment be prescribed?
  (5) Should all patients with symptoms suggesting infection
      be treated?
  (6) Is there any need for follow-up?
  (7) Should radiological investigation be ordered in some/all
      men from general practice?

(8) Which patients should be referred to hospital, to what sort of specialist and for what purpose?

Chapter Four *Urinary Tract Infection in Childhood*

Questions
  (1) Under what circumstances should we consider the possibility of urinary tract infection in a child?
  (2) How should we examine the patient?
  (3) Do we need a urine specimen and how should we obtain it?
  (4) How many specimens should we obtain before starting treatment or referral?
  (5) What drugs should we use and for how long should they be taken?
  (6) What can we say to the parents?
  (7) Can we say anything useful to the child?
  (8) Do we refer all cases to a specialist?
  (9) If not, how do we select patients for referral?
 (10) To what sort of specialist should we refer children with infection and why?
 (11) Is follow-up necessary?
 (12) Should we allow the hospital to take over follow-up?
 (13) What are the minimum facilities needed to ensure adequate follow-up at least some of the time in general practice?
 (14) How should a follow-up consultation be conducted and for how long should follow-up continue?
 (15) Is screening necessary/desirable/a waste of resources?

Chapter Five *Urinary Tract Infection and the Elderly*

Questions
  (1) What problems do the elderly have in relation to urinary tract infection?
  (2) What should we look for in the history?
  (3) When do we need to and how do we examine old people with urinary tract infection?

(4) Is bacterial assessment of the urine necessary?
(5) What drug treatment should we give?
(6) Do we need to refer old people with infection to hospital?
(7) Should they be followed up afterwards?
(8) What are the risks of infection with indwelling catheters?

D. BROOKS

1

CONCEPTS, DEFINITIONS AND THEIR PRACTICAL VALUE – AN OVERVIEW

D. BROOKS

A GLOSSARY OF TERMS

In his book published in 1976 Henrik Wulff argued that in order to make rational clinical decisions it is necessary to make a diagnosis – but a diagnosis he said is not an end in itself, merely a mental resting place for prognostic considerations and therapeutic decision[1]. In order to establish a diagnosis two conditions need to be fulfilled. First it is necessary to examine the various manifestations of disease in the patient. Secondly one must be familiar with the nosological description of a number of diseases. It is then possible to decide which disease description best fits the collected data and to find the name of the disease representing the diagnosis.

If we are to achieve these we must know what we are talking about. The Medical Research Council has produced a number of definitions which it is hoped will aid both the diagnostic

1

process and the search for new knowledge and new standards. These are listed here and are followed by other terms in common use.

Medical Research Council definitions

Urinary tract infection The presence of micro-organisms within the urinary tract.

Bacteriuria The presence of bacteria in bladder urine. For epidemiological purposes this may be detected by quantitative urine culture; its presence is usually indicated by the finding of $\geqslant 100\,000$ colony forming units (c.f.u.) per ml of freshly voided urine and any growth from urine obtained by suprapubic aspiration.

Bladder bacteriuria The presence of bacteria in urine obtained by suprapubic aspiration.

Covert bacteriuria Significant bacteriuria detected by the screening of apparently healthy populations. The use of this term is preferred to asymptomatic bacteriuria (which is still widely used).

Upper-tract bacteriuria The presence of bacteria in urine collected from the renal pelvis or ureter(s) or both. This may indicate renal infection but in the presence of vesico-ureteric reflux the organisms may derive from the bladder.

Frequency and dysuria syndrome A clinical syndrome often called cystitis (especially by lay people) consisting of frequency and dysuria. Bladder bacteriuria may or may not be present.

Bacterial cystitis A syndrome consisting of dysuria and frequency of micturition by day and night. Bladder bacteriuria is present and is usually associated with pyuria and sometimes haematuria.

Abacterial cystitis A syndrome consisting of frequency and dysuria in the absence of bladder bacteriuria. The use of the term urethral syndrome is not recommended because there is no evidence of urethral disease in most of the patients.

Acute bacterial pyelonephritis A syndrome consisting of loin pain, loin tenderness and pyrexia accompanied by bacteriuria, bacteraemia, pyuria and sometimes haematuria. The condition is associated with bacterial infection of the kidney.

Response to treatment Disappearance of bacteriuria after treatment.

Relapse Post treatment recurrence of bacteriuria due to the same organism as that originally isolated. Relapse of infection usually occurs within six weeks of cessation of treatment.

Persistant infection Bacteriuria persisting during and after treatment.

Reinfection Recurrence of bacteriuria after treatment due to an organism different from that originally isolated. Reinfection with the same organism cannot be differentiated from relapse.

Criteria for cure In all treatment trials these should be carefully defined. Urine specimens should be collected at specified times after completion of treatment over a defined period (usually not less than six weeks). If the post treatment specimens show a relapse or the bacteriuria persists treatment may be deemed to have failed.

Other terms in common use

Dysuria Used to describe painful and/or difficult micturition. The pain may be suprapubic, pelvic aching or a burning sensation in the urethra or urethral orifice. All may occur only during micturition or may be virtually constant throughout an episode of infection.

Frequency This is said to occur when the amount of urine

passed is consistently less than the capacity of the normal bladder, which is about 300–500 ml. Most people urinate every 3–4 h during the day and perhaps once at night. Frequency of micturition represents altered bladder function (as opposed to polyuria which represents altered renal function) and usually accompanies acute inflammation.

Urgency There is a strong desire to empty the bladder which may be powerful enough to overcome sphincter control and lead to urgency incontinence.

Strangury This term is used when difficult and painful micturition is accompanied by spasms of the pelvic musculature.

Prostatism This is a symptom complex characterized by hesitancy or delay in initiating micturition, interruption of the urine stream and decreased force and calibre of the urinary stream. The commonest cause is prostate hypertrophy.

Pyuria Presence of abnormal numbers of leucocytes in urine. The number of urinary leucocytes which can be regarded as normal depends crucially on the method of assessment. In a centrifuged specimen (5 min at 750 g) the upper limit of leucocytes[2] in a carefully collected specimen is 2000 ml^{-1} or 200 000 h^{-1}. The leucocyte excretion rate is a more accurate measurement but it is more difficult to measure. Pyuria represents tissue involvement which is not necessarily present in all patients with bacteriuria and may be due to other inflammatory causes. Vaginal leucocytes can easily contaminate a specimen.

Chronic pyelonephritis Macroscopically the kidneys are scarred and possibly unequal in size and shape. On cut section scars may run from cortex to medulla and the calyces may be dilated and deformed.

On microscopic examination there is evidence of a focal inflammatory reaction primarily involving the interstitial tissue in the medulla but also extending into the cortex. Fibrosis varies according to the inflammatory process and blood vessels, tubules and glomeruli may be secondarily involved in this.

For many years it was believed that these features were the result of chronic bacterial inflammation but it is now considered that many other non-bacterial processes might produce them. These include renal artery stenosis, urinary tract obstruction, renal arteriosclerosis, drug allergy and analgesic abuse. The changes have been associated with ascending urinary tract infection and vesico-ureteric reflux in infancy and early childhood.

Vesico-ureteric reflux This term describes reflux of urine through an incomplete vesico-ureteric valve from the bladder into the ureter. The condition is defined on the basis of cystography performed during micturition. Reflux has been graded though grading can be difficult due to varying states of hydration.

Grade I: contrast medium enters the ureter during micturition but does not reach the pelvis.

Grade II: contrast medium reaches the pelvis but does not cause distension of the pelvi-calyceal system.

Grade III: the pelvi-calyceal system is distended by contrast medium which refluxes during micturition.

Any general practitioner hoping to improve our understanding of these common conditions will need a working understanding of these definitions – how else can experiences be shared? However, it is not necessarily perverse to question, as we sometimes do in this book, their relevance to daily clinical practice.

Organisms that may be involved in urinary tract infection

The organisms that are isolated from urinary tract infections are those that are prevalent in the bowel flora. Table 1.1 lists these organisms and compares a typical general practice series with a typical hospital series. It will be noticed that there are differences. *Escherichia coli* tends to be commoner in general practice. This illustrates the selective effect of the referral process on the study of the aetiology of a disease. Many strains of *Staphylococcus albus* when examined by the Baird-Parker technique[3] are resistant to novobiocin and are often referred to as type three micrococci. These also are prevalent in the bowel flora but they have been found to have the highest incidence in young women, suggesting a possible relationship with intercourse-induced infection. It is of interest that they share with *Proteus mirabilis* the distinction of being the second commonest organism in general practice in this series. *Pseudomonas pyocyanea* is rarely found unless there has been instrumentation of the genito-urinary tract or there are abnormalities such as large renal calculi or urinary tract obstruction.

Table 1.1   Urinary pathogens in general practice and in hospital practice during 1977 (as percentage of total infections)

General practice	Organisms	Hospital practice
73.1	*Escherichia coli*	40.9
6.0	*Staphylococcus albus*	6.5
5.7	*Proteus mirabilis*	10.8
4.8	*Klebsiella*	13.6
3.4	*Streptococcus faecalis*	12.1
3.0	*Enterobacter* (*Citrobacter* spp.)	3.9
1.4	*Pseudomonas pyocyanea*	4.8
0.9	*Streptococci* (non-faecal)	2.2
0.7	*Proteus vulgaris*	2.0
0.4	*Staphylococcus aureus* (coag-ulase positive)	2.5
0.4	Others	0.6

Figures supplied by kind permission of Dr S. J. Eykyn, Department of Clinical Microbiology, St Thomas's Hospital, London. Based on 2110 hospitals and 435 general practice infection episodes.

Bacterial aetiology does, however, vary with age and sex. There is, for example, a predominance of *Proteus* species in boys over 12 months old. An important finding (which first appeared from general practice) was that only one half of women who consult their doctors because they are suffering from acute dysuria and frequency of micturition have significant bacteriuria. Until recently the term urethral syndrome was used to describe this group though we are now advised to use the term abacterial cystitis. The cause of the symptoms is puzzling and while some authors have advocated that conventional organisms in low numbers are responsible[4] others have incriminated organisms such as *Chlamydia*, herpes, *Trichomonas* and *Gardnerella*. Organisms with fastidious growth requirements such as *Lactobacilli* spp. *Streptococcus milleri* and *Corynebacterium* spp. have also been blamed[5]. No one view has achieved general recognition.

Viruses and the urinary tract

Viruria is commonly observed during systemic virus infections caused by, for example, rubella, cytomegalovirus, measles, mumps, vaccinia, herpes simplex and Coxsackie species. However, this phenomenon is thought to be due to shedding of virus from kidney cells involved in the generalized infection, or even by glomerular filtration. It is believed to be harmless although occasionally mild transitory impairment of renal function has been observed. Certainly viruria is not associated with symptoms suggesting urinary tract infection, and attempts to identify viruses in such patients when bacteria cannot be identified have usually been unsuccessful.

In 1973 Japanese workers[6] identified adenovirus type II in 11 out of 28 consecutive children who complained of acute haematuria, dysuria and frequency and did not have bacteriuria; in nine of the 17 patients with acute haemorrhagic 'cystitis' of childhood who did not have viruria a specific antibody response was demonstrated. The condition is commoner in boys and is believed to be benign. Herpes simplex type II has been incriminated in the aetiology of some types of prostatitis but the evidence for this is not yet substantial enough to be conclusive.

As far as chronic renal disease is concerned, there has been speculation that viruses might produce chronic pyelonephritis and glomerulonephritis is sometimes caused by an immune complex disease involving viral antigens.

Tuberculosis

Infection of the urogenital tract with *Mycobacterium tuberculosis* is rare in general practice. However, it should be suspected where there is persistent sterile pyuria. In the male, infection usually involves kidney and bladder, prostate, epididymis and testicle together. In the female, the Fallopian tubes may be infected. Symptoms are usually insidious with abdominal discomfort and specific genito-urinary complaints.

Other organisms

A clinical picture similar to that of acute bacterial infection may be produced by fungal infection of the urogenital tract and various species may be involved including *Candida* which grows well in urine and can be cultured from it. Fungus infections are also rare in general practice; patients usually have other problems such as diabetes mellitus or neoplasm, or are on long-term antibiotic therapy.

A MODEL OF POSSIBLE MECHANISMS FOR THE PATHOGENESIS OF ASCENDING INFECTION IN THE URINARY TRACT

Urinary tract infections may best be thought of as a continuous process beginning in the urethra and progressing to the bladder. Once the bladder urine is infected it is possible to argue that organisms might ascend to the renal parenchyma and produce acute pyelonephritis. The pathogenesis of this process is not well understood but in children, at least, failure of the normal vesico-ureteric valve mechanisms to develop (and in adults temporary or permanent failure to function) is believed to play an important part.

Figure 1.1 is a model of possible mechanisms by which infection may ascend the urinary tract. It can be envisaged as a step-by-step overcoming of the natural defences. Ascending infection is believed to be the usual mode of infection but the urinary tract is normally resistant to infection. Self-evidently, for example, all women have potential pathogens in the bowel flora yet not all women develop UTI.

Defence of the urinary tract

The first line of defence (Figure 1.1) is opposition to pathogen colonization by commensals on the perineum and vestibule, in women, and in the distal urethra; swabs taken from these locations reveal a varied flora.

If pathogens do colonize the urethra the next defence (this is the single most effective defence against ascending infection) is the normal voiding of the urine. This is also the major defence of the bladder itself if pathogens enter the bladder urine.

It has been demonstrated in volunteers that the diluting effect of ureteric urine and frequent bladder emptying, and the flushing effect of urine passing down the urethra remove bacteria introduced into the bladder under experimental conditions. Urine itself is thought to be a good culture medium

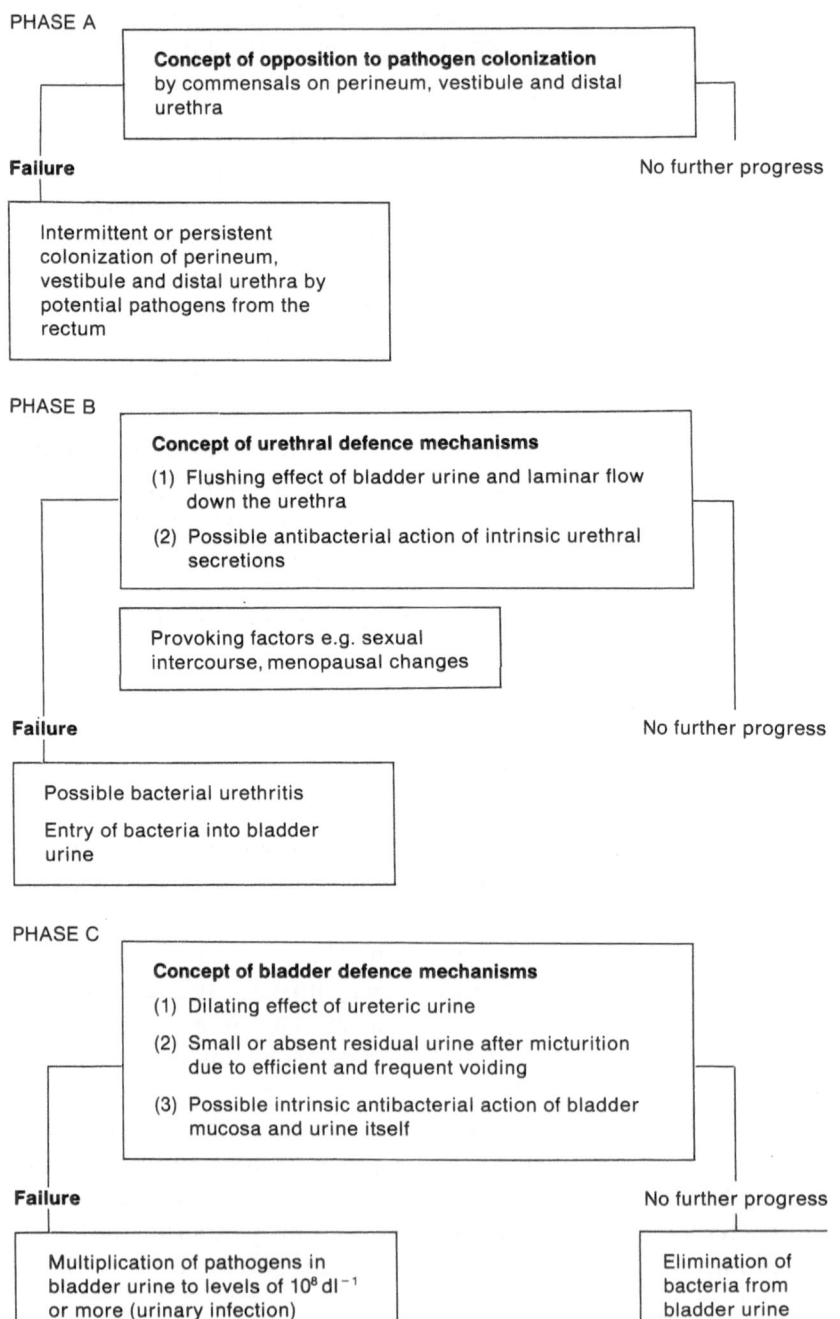

PHASE A

Concept of opposition to pathogen colonization
by commensals on perineum, vestibule and distal
urethra

Failure   No further progress

Intermittent or persistent
colonization of perineum,
vestibule and distal urethra by
potential pathogens from the
rectum

PHASE B

Concept of urethral defence mechanisms

(1) Flushing effect of bladder urine and laminar flow
down the urethra

(2) Possible antibacterial action of intrinsic urethral
secretions

Provoking factors e.g. sexual
intercourse, menopausal changes

Failure   No further progress

Possible bacterial urethritis

Entry of bacteria into bladder
urine

PHASE C

Concept of bladder defence mechanisms

(1) Dilating effect of ureteric urine

(2) Small or absent residual urine after micturition
due to efficient and frequent voiding

(3) Possible intrinsic antibacterial action of bladder
mucosa and urine itself

Failure   No further progress

Multiplication of pathogens in
bladder urine to levels of $10^8 \, dl^{-1}$
or more (urinary infection)

Elimination of
bacteria from
bladder urine

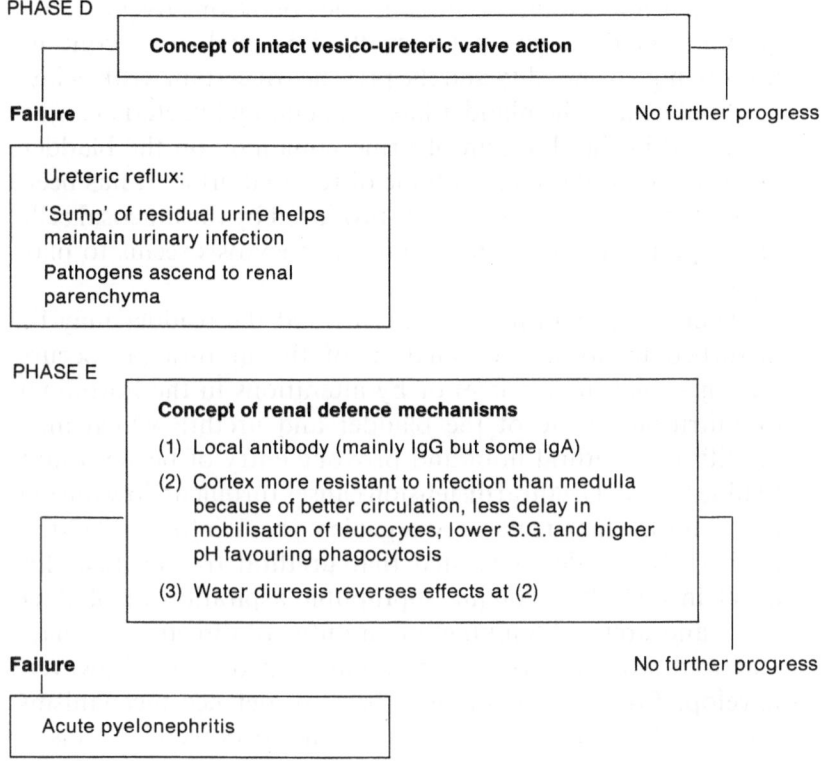

PHASE D

Concept of intact vesico-ureteric valve action

Failure   No further progress

Ureteric reflux:

'Sump' of residual urine helps
maintain urinary infection

Pathogens ascend to renal
parenchyma

PHASE E

Concept of renal defence mechanisms

(1) Local antibody (mainly IgG but some IgA)

(2) Cortex more resistant to infection than medulla
    because of better circulation, less delay in
    mobilisation of leucocytes, lower S.G. and higher
    pH favouring phagocytosis

(3) Water diuresis reverses effects at (2)

Failure   No further progress

Acute pyelonephritis

Figure 1.1   Possible mechanisms for the pathogenesis of ascending infection within the urinary tract: a step-by-step failure of natural defences

but this is not always so. Favourable conditions for bacterial growth include a low pH (usually 5.5), high urea concentration, high osmolality and the presence of certain weak acids. Normally when the bladder has been emptied bacteria can be destroyed in the thin film of urine remaining on the bladder mucosa and in the small volume of residual urine. It has been suggested that the organic acids produced by the mucosal cells are responsible for this effect but phagocytosis seems to play a part.

Defence mechanisms in the urine and the bladder may be disturbed by local manipulation of the urethra (as occurs during sexual intercourse) or by alterations in the hormonal or nutritional state of the bladder and urethra which may modify the urethral flora and provoke entry of bacteria into bladder urine. Urethral distension causes turbulent flow during micturition which may carry organisms back into the bladder. In 1975 Kaye[7] demonstrated that urethral trauma had this effect in a study involving suprapubic aspiration of bladder urine and urethral 'milking' in an outward direction in anaesthetized women; urinary tract infection did not, however, develop. Presumably this was because defence mechanisms removed the organisms while their numbers were still insignificant.

Invasion of the renal parenchyma is the last phase in the progressive ascent of infection of the urinary tract; each advance of the pathogens being of escalating importance to the patient. The kidney is protected by the vesico-ureteral valve. When the action of this valve is faulty vesico-ureteral reflux creates a 'sump' of residual urine in which pathogens may flourish and from which they can ascend to the kidney. This may also be the outcome when residual urine is the result of obstruction or neurological disease.

Bacterial invasion of the renal tissue usually involves the medulla rather than the cortex, for reasons which include poor circulation in the medulla, higher specific gravity and lower pH, all of which tend to impair phagocytosis. It is believed that bacteria can ascend to the kidney in the absence of reflux by simple Brownian movement, and experimental evidence suggests that the lymphatic channels may be involved; blood borne infection is believed to be uncommon except in infants.

The clinical picture

The clinical picture will reflect the stage of infection. In a small group of women recurrent symptoms may be produced solely by non-infective factors and pathogens might never enter the urinary tract. In others, bacterial urethritis, where precipitating factors may have weakened urethral defence mechanisms, would not be associated with organisms in mid-stream specimens of urine. A larger group might alternate between bacterial urethritis and bladder urine infection (which occurs when organisms enter and multiply in the bladder) depending on the severity of the precipitating factors and the consequent state of the natural defence mechanisms. Finally there would be a group in whom bladder urine infection might always occur when bacteria invaded the urethra.

Precipitating factors

Sexual intercourse

A relationship between sexual intercourse and lower urinary tract symptoms in women was first reported by Rovsing in 1897[8]. In 1965 the urologists Moore and Hira[9] questioned 182 women at an out-patient clinic and found that 11 per cent admitted that intercourse was a precipitating factor. In 1972 Brooks and Maudar[4] in a general practice study reported that the frequency and dysuria syndrome was precipitated by sexual intercourse in 30 per cent of women, when bacteriuria was isolated, and in 20 per cent of women in the absence of bacteriuria and that this relationship was particularly noticeable in younger women.

Cold weather

It is common clinical experience to find that patients with urinary symptoms relate their onset to cold weather; Moore and Hira found this to be the case with 5 per cent of women. Brooks and Maudar gave a similar report for 15 per cent of women with dysuria and frequency and bacteriuria and 30 per cent of women with symptoms and low organism counts; they also found that nearly twice as many presented during the three months September to November as presented during the three previous months.

Emotional disturbance

About 16 per cent of women with acute dysuria and frequency notice a relationship between the onset of symptoms and emotional stress, whether or not bacteriuria is present, and from his knowledge of them the practitioner may recognize those women who are vulnerable to stress.

Catheterization

In 1879 Sir Henry Thomson[10] described the development of cystitis by contagion through the use of instruments. He referred to a doctor with the daily habit of using a silver catheter on himself who on one occasion used the catheter on another person. This person subsequently developed a mucopurulent urine associated with dysuria and mild rigor. Thomson postulated the existence of infectious material in the crevices of the catheter; an alternative explanation would involve urethral trauma and impairment of defence mechanisms. In 1956 Kass[11] calculated that infection followed in about 2 per cent of cases of catheterization. In 1972 Brooks and Maudar[4] found that one third of women with symptoms recalled past catheterization on one or more occasions, whether or not they had bacteriuria. Eighteen per cent had a history of cervical dilation and curettage and 8 per cent had had a hysterectomy; others had received surgery for prolapse repair, cone biopsy and other gynaecological procedures. In all cases catheterization had been performed.

About 6 per cent of women blamed gynaecological surgery directly for the onset of recurrent attacks; in five women the syndrome followed within one week of gynaecological procedures in which catheterization was performed. It is obvious that indications for routine catheterization in gynaecological practice are in need of reassessment.

Allergy

In 1949 Kindall and Nickells[12] stated that allergy in the urinary tract was frequently unrecognized. However, by 1972 Brooks and Maudar could report[4] five patients in whom allergic mechanisms may have played a part in the development of symptoms. Two of them had dysuria and frequency and also bacteriuria; of these one reported that wearing nylon underwear produced attacks, the other (who had eosinophilia) blamed the local use of an aerosol deodorant. The three patients without bacteriuria blamed eggs and citrus fruits; one who blamed eggs for the production of symptoms had an eosinophil count of 1760 per mm^3 during the acute episode.

The menopause and autonomic ageing

Most general practitioners will recall patients who developed the frequency and dysuria syndrome during the menopause or in whom these symptoms became worse at this time. Alterations in the urethral mucosa similar to those occurring in the vagina may well modify defence mechanisms. Brocklehurst et al.[13] emphasized that in older women, because of neurogenic change and/or outlet obstruction, the bladder neither fills nor empties properly and as a result a constant 'sump' of residual urine is present, which interferes with normal bladder defence mechanisms.

Other factors

A few women will cite menstruation, bubble baths, pregnancy, bouts of diarrhoea, upper respiratory tract infections and pressure on the urethra from tampons as the cause of the frequency and dysuria syndrome; such associations are difficult to prove. But it is probable that as yet unrecognized factors may interfere with defence mechanisms and allow bowel flora to ascend the urethra and become established in the bladder urine; oral contraceptives and intrauterine devices are obvious suspects.

BACTERIURIA

The term abacterial cystitis describes the presence of symptoms without bladder bacteriuria. These patients have received much attention; whether bacteria are involved or not is in dispute. Many workers believe that the syndrome is caused by acute or chronic bacterial infection of the urethral mucosa, possibly involving Skenes glands. Bladder bacteriuria cannot be expected in such cases. However, workers at St Bartholomew's Hospital have been unable to establish the presence of inflammatory change in the urethral mucosa or lumen narrowing. They claim that nearly two-thirds of women referred with symptoms and not having bacteriuria on the first attendance develop a bacteriuria on a 9-month follow-up. But they do also point out that some never develop bacteriuria, and that there is no evidence of bacterial involvement in the production of symptoms in this group. The natural history of this condition remains uncertain.

Tapsall and his colleagues have speculated[14] that nearly

all urinary infection might be asymptomatic, and that the frequency and dysuria syndrome is not caused by bacteria at all but by those various precipitating factors which as well as causing symptoms impair defence mechanisms; bacteriuria, in this view, is an inevitable but silent consequence. Bacteria would then be significant pathogens only in the small proportion of cases which did not resolve spontaneously as the insult to the defence mechanisms subsided.

A criterion established by Kass (see below) has been widely used to discriminate between those levels of bacteriuria thought to be of diagnostic significance and those that are not. It seems to me, as it does to Tapsall and his colleagues, that the separation of women with dysuria and frequency into two groups solely on the basis of significant bacteriuria is not as helpful in management or prognosis as was once thought. Kass's criterion produces an arbitrary division; if bacteria are important in a proportion of patients (who might be helped by antibacterial therapy) the Kass criterion does not necessarily identify them.

The bacteriological count

Much of our modern understanding of the bacteriology of urinary tract infection is based upon the work of Professor Edward Kass of the Department of Bacteriology and Immunology at Harvard Medical School. In 1956, although attempts to identify chronic pyelonephritis in patients with urinary infection had not been particularly successful, a close aetiological relationship was widely suspected. Kass concentrated his attention on patients with asymptomatic urinary infection which was not easy to diagnose bacteriologically because there were no generally accepted criteria for differentiating true urinary infection (i.e. the multiplication of bacteria within bladder urine) from accidental contamination during micturition.

Organisms that cause urinary tract infection are those prevalent in the bowel flora and therefore they may be present on the perineum or in the distal urethra. They may enter the urine during micturition even in cases where there is no infection within the urinary tract in terms of multiplication within bladder urine or tissue invasion in the urethra. This is termed contamination and should be distinguished from colonization which occurs in the first stage of an ascending urinary infection.

Kass carried out *in vitro* experiments which demonstrated that bacteria introduced into pooled sterile urine specimens multiplied rapidly to numbers of organisms of about $10^{11} l^{-1}$ within an hour or so. This should similarly occur *in vivo* in the bladder urine, he argued, and from experimental studies on large numbers of asymptomatic and symptomatic patients he concluded that if bacteria were multiplying in the bladder urine the count would usually be $10^8 l^{-1}$ or more; conversely a count of $10^7 l^{-1}$ or less was nearly always the result of contamination, as bacterial multiplication could not have occurred in bladder urine. On the rare occasions that counts between 10^7 and $10^8 l^{-1}$ were obtained the result was regarded as equivocal and the investigation was repeated.

This concept of a diagnostically significant level of bacteriuria had been widely accepted for many years (the idea that all counts below $10^8 l^{-1}$ were contamination has now been discarded), although Kass himself emphasized that anything interfering with bacterial multiplication in the bladder urine, such as the presence of antibiotics in the urine or marked frequency of micturition, could result in lower counts assuming significance. However, it is now realized that Kass's work has more fundamental limitations. We are less certain that urine is always a good culture medium and that all organisms multiply at the same rate. Furthermore gram-positive cocci tend to be under represented in colony counts compared with gram-negative bacilli. The possibility of urinary tract infection distal to the bladder in the urethra must also be considered, since, if tissue invasion has occurred in the urethra, the possibility of multiplication in bladder urine does not exist.

Kass emphasized that urine at room temperature needed to be examined within an hour if significant multiplication of contaminant was to be avoided. This requirement proved an almost insurmountable difficulty in active family practices until new techniques were developed to overcome the problem. To be acceptable for routine use a test must not only be sensitive – earlier chemical tests identified high bacterial counts indiscriminately without distinguishing pathogens from non-pathogens – but simple and reliable enough for the general practitioner to use. Only two methods are now recommended: the boric acid preservation of urine samples and the dip inoculation technique.

The boric acid method has the advantage that microscopical examination of the specimen can be carried out in the laboratory. The dip inoculation technique is particularly adaptable to the needs of the general practitioner because incubation can be undertaken on the surgery premises giving a rapid and reliable estimation of the bacterial content of the urine specimen. It has been demonstrated that general practitioners are just as accurate in interpreting dipslides as hospital bacteriologists. However, specimens from family practice give reliable results even when posted to the laboratory.

Figures 1.2 and 1.3 show Tillotts dipslides with organism counts indicating significant bacteriuria and contamination, respectively. One side of the slide is coated with MacConkey agar and the other side is coated with cystine–lactose electrolyte-deficient (CLED) medium. MacConkey medium was originally designed for work with gram-negative organisms from the gut, and its ability to support the growth of gram-positive urinary pathogens is notoriously variable. CLED medium supports the growth of all commonly encountered pathogens and is preferred by many bacteriologists. If incubation is carried out on the practice premises the positive slides can be posted to the laboratory for drug sensitivity tests, should these be required. Unfortunately at the time of writing dipslides are not yet generally available in family practice but the Public Health Laboratories supply them on request and

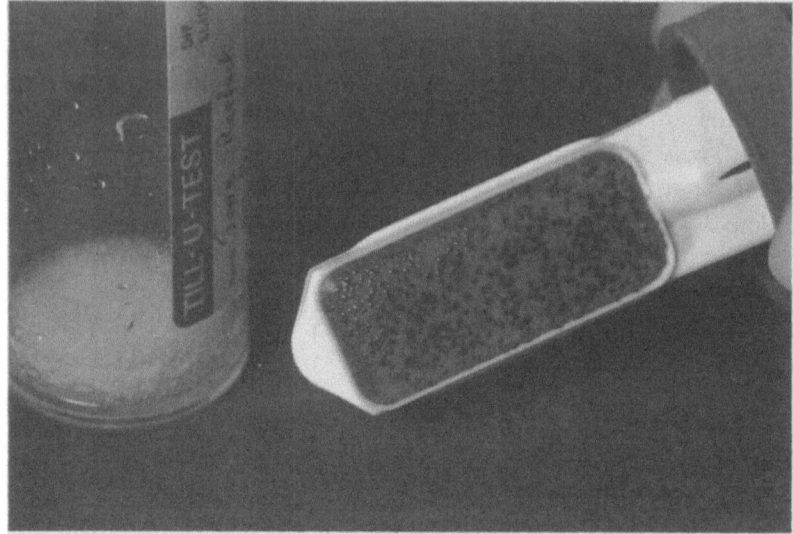

Figure 1.2   Significant bacteriuria on a Till-U-Test dipslide

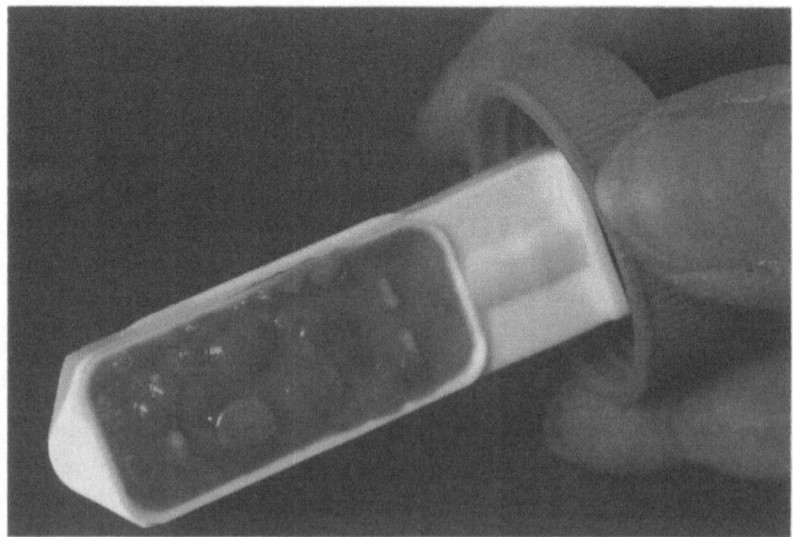

Figure 1.3   'Contamination' on a Till-U-Test dipslide

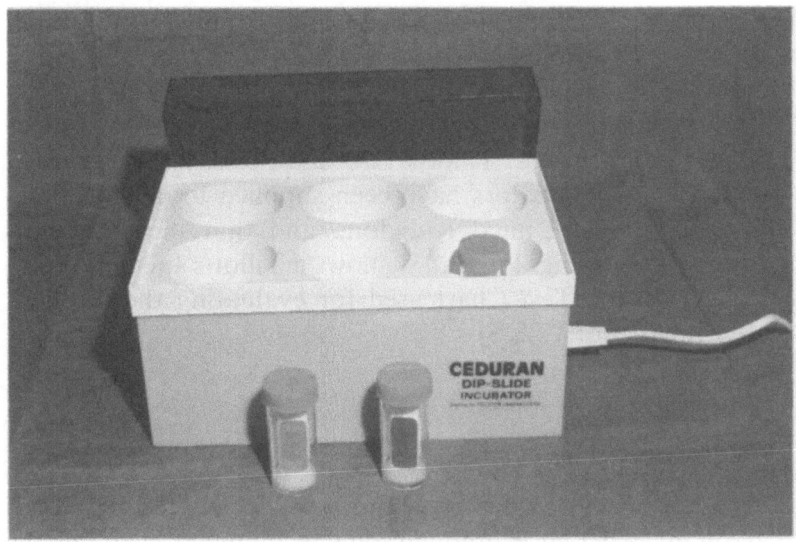

Figure 1.4   A Tillott's Incubator for practice use

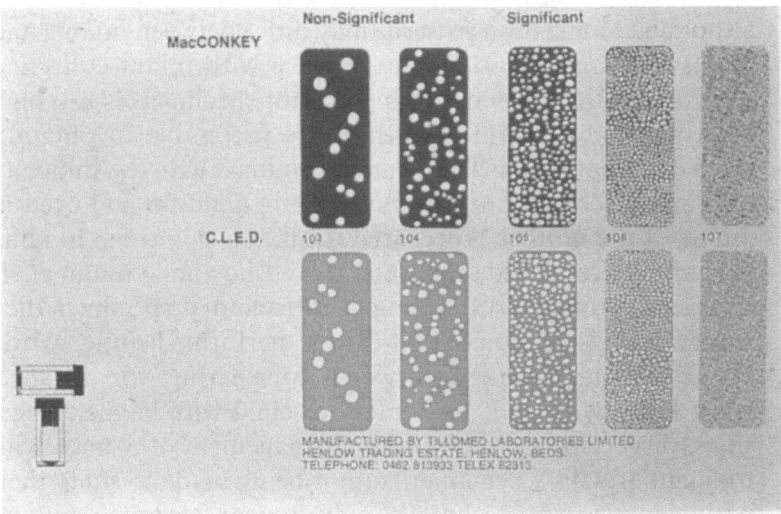

Figure 1.5   A Test Chart used to assess the concentration of organisms in a urine specimen

many District Health Authorities will distribute them through hospital bacteriology departments. A word of caution – occasionally water may be lost from the medium during storage leaving a desiccated membrane on the slide; such slides should be discarded. Tillotts Laboratories say that approximately 4000 incubators have been supplied to general practitioners in the United Kingdom, and that the number is steadily increasing. Figure 1.4 shows a Tillotts Incubator and Figure 1.5 the Test Chart used for evaluating the dipslides after incubation.

Collection of a specimen

Preparation of the adult patient does not appear to be necessary in my experience although some recommend swabbing the perineum with cotton wool moistened with tap water. For infants or young children however swabbing may be recommended since the incidence of contaminated specimens is higher due, I suspect, to the absence of bladder control, although colonization patterns may differ between infants and adults (see Chapter 4). My experience with infant collecting bags is that the incidence of high count specimens is too high at around 60 per cent, and that it is preferable to obtain a clean catch specimen. These can be obtained with less difficulty than might be imagined in most young children and even in infants if the mother is prepared to sit in a side room holding her infant over a wide-mouthed waxed hospital container. If there are problems in getting a satisfactory specimen then suprapubic aspiration (SPA) can be performed quite swiftly in the surgery. This is well worth considering, for instance, when faced with an ill and fractious child with vague clinical signs, or very occasionally in the management of women with frequent attacks when an attempt is being made to study their pathogenesis. The technique may appear alarming but on reflection is no more hazardous than a venepuncture, and many thousands of specimens have now been obtained in this way without mishap. Even when bowel contents have been aspirated the patient has been none the worse for the experience! After preliminary swabbing with ether the urine is obtained with a 10 ml syringe and an intravenous needle: entry is made about 2.5 cm above the symphysis in the mid-line. My experience, solely with infants, has been an overall success rate of about 50 per cent. If the napkin is dry and the bladder palpable the success rate is much higher. It is probably advisable to anaesthetize the skin in adults.

CLINICAL DIAGNOSIS AND MANAGEMENT

An overview

Our knowledge of the nature, course and outcome of any disease process will obviously depend upon the study in patients of the development of symptoms and signs over a period of time. A parallel record of changes in appropriate scientific parameters (whether biochemical, histopathological or immunological) further defines the aetiology and pathogenesis of the underlying disease and knowledge gained in this way is then used to produce diagnostic criteria and management norms which can be recommended and supported for use in clinical practice.

However, the division of medical care into primary care and secondary or hospital care systems has inevitably had a significant effect; knowledge and clinical standards gained by study of one population cannot necessarily be applied to another unless bias introduced by population selection can be excluded with certainty. This concept is of particular relevance in the study of urinary tract infection which is primarily a community problem. Only 10 per cent of women with symptoms bother to consult a doctor and less than 10 per cent of the patients seen by the general practitioner are referred to hospital specialists (Table 1.2). In the past, confident statements about the prognosis of this disease process have been made supported only by studies on hospital patients and these

Table 1.2 Percentage from general practice of patients with cystitis and pyelonephritis

Clinical diagnosis	Action taken by general practitioner		
	Admission to hospital	Out-patient referral or domicillary visit	Laboratory investigation
Cystitis	0.5	3.4	43.4
Pyelonephritis	1.7	6.3	55.6

Sources: DHSS *Morbidity statistics from general practice* (1970–71). London, HMSO; Office of Population Census and Surveys; the RCGP (1974).

have not always proved accurate. For example, we now know that there is no evidence that repeated attacks of dysuria and frequency in women lead to kidney failure. The assumption of kidney failure was based on hospital experience; although general practitioners did not find evidence to support the assumption, hospital experience led us to believe otherwise. Even the aetiology of urinary infection can vary between hospital and general practice as a result of the referral process, as Table 1.2 illustrates.

If they are to be effective, diagnostic criteria and management norms for general practice must be supported by the experience of general practice. Here is an example: an approach recently described by a hospital specialist, for the management of women with dysuria and frequency syndrome in general practice, comprised a careful history, physical examination (including a pelvic examination), a precise bacteriological diagnosis and a high vaginal swab to exclude gonorrhoea. This kind of approach is far more helpful for managing hospital patients; these detailed recommendations are based on experience of patients with very frequent or atypical symptoms who had been referred for a second opinion.

As recently as 1986 a provocative suggestion came from a hospital that '... a postal survey claims that 94 per cent of practitioners start treatment before receiving laboratory reports and only 14 per cent stop treatment if the result is negative. If this is what happens country-wide it represents wastage of public funds on a large scale[15]. Can this truly be what is happening?

General practitioners vary considerably in their use of laboratory services. The reasons for this are largely unknown but there is some evidence that those who are more recently qualified make greater use of the laboratory. A recent Public Health Laboratory survey showed that the overall ratio of hospital urine specimens examined to general practice specimens is nearly 3:1 and that only one-third of general practitioners actually send urine specimens for more than 80 per cent of patients with suspected urinary infection compared with nearly all consultants[16]. Nearly half the patients presenting with symptoms in practices participating in the National Morbidity Survey received bacteriological investigation. Both these studies probably overestimate usage of the laboratory by general practitioners, as the Public Health Laboratory survey was biased in favour of doctors who actually use the laboratory, and the National Morbidity Survey selected more efficient and possibly better practices, with principals younger than the national average. Paradoxically, 90 per cent of patients with urinary tract infections are dealt with entirely by the general practitioner himself, only a small minority being referred for a specialist opinion. These observations pose a number of intriguing questions.

(1) How reliable (or useful) is a clinical diagnosis of urinary infection as a 'mental resting place' (in Wulff's terms[1]) for therapy and prognosis?

(2) Does the selection and screening of patients before they reach hospital doctors alter the aetiology, diagnosis, management and prognosis in a hospital population compared with a general practice population – thereby altering the need for bacteriological assessment?

(3) Should patients with symptoms be investigated bac-

teriologically in or from general practice? If so, is this because urinary tract infection should be taken seriously and reliable evidence of its presence is essential if the right patients are to be referred to specialists? Or is it because therapeutic intervention is a serious matter and reliable information is needed to avoid subjecting patients unnecessarily to drug treatments?

(4) Are general practitioners under-investigating patients with urinary infection and are hospital doctors over-investigating them?

There is no doubt that the low usage of the laboratory service by general practitioners partly reflects their isolation from clinical and laboratory colleagues when the National Health Service was introduced in 1948. The practical difficulties of getting urine examined may also have encouraged the development of attitudes, about the significance of urinary tract infection, in general practitioners that differed from those of hospital doctors, especially based as it has been on experience with a different denominator population. And, of course, the practical difficulties may in themselves militate against frequent use of the laboratory service inasmuch as they may cause considerable operational difficulties. Delays in collecting a specimen, its transportation to the laboratory, and the time taken in awaiting the report on it may create considerable operational problems. Many patients – particularly the very young and very old – are seen at home and they may be too ill to attend the laboratory which, of course, may not be open at a convenient time. This leads us to the community-aspect of general practice.

General practice in the community

If we are to derive diagnostic criteria and management norms for ourselves and set standards for care in general practice, we cannot do this without considering the role of the general

Table 1.3   The general practitioner: a job definition

The General Practitioner is a licenced medical graduate who gives personal primary and continuing care to individuals, families and a practice population irrespective of age, sex and illness. It is the synthesis of these functions which is unique. He will attend his patients in his consulting room and in their homes and sometimes in a clinic or hospital. His aim is to make early diagnosis. He will include and integrate physical, psychological and social factors in his considerations about health and illness. This will be expressed in the care of his patients. He will make an initial decision about every problem which is presented to him as a doctor. He will undertake the continuing management of his patients with chronic, recurrent or terminal illnesses. Prolonged contact means that he can use repeated opportunities to gather information at a pace appropriate to each patient and build up a relationship of trust which he can use professionally. He will practise in co-operation with other colleagues, medical and non-medical. He will know how and when to intervene through treatment, prevention and education to promote the health of his patients and their families. He will recognize that he also has a professional responsibility to the community.

practitioner in the community (Table 1.3). Society requires direct and easy access to a low cost non-hierarchical system of care provided by a primary health care team with skills which can be readily adapted to the needs of the community. Above all, continuing responsibility and the personal professional relationship between a general practitioner and his patient demand that physical, psychological and social factors should be built into any behavioural statement we might produce.

In this context it is difficult to improve on the words of Professor Kass who accused the profession of being too disease-oriented because we consider urinary tract infection only in terms of renal failure.

'The effect of bacteriuria as a cause of absence from school or from work needs more direct measurement. Observations on the absentee records of schoolgirls during the years preceding the discovery of their bacteriuria would be a useful approach to determining whether bacteriuria had an adverse affect on daily lives. It is more difficult to gauge the emotional impact of the teaching that sexual activity is a determinant of bacteriuria. One suspects that there is more personal unhappiness and marital discord arising from this teaching than is immediately obvious. The key point is that we address ourselves to determining the impact of chronic disorders such as bacteriuria on a broader life experience and not limit ourselves to one or other selected end-point that happens to be of particular interest.'

The eminent bacteriologist who gave his name to the concept of significant bacteriuria thus supports ideas which embody current thinking about general practice.

But what of the patients' views? General practitioners deal largely with women with the dysuria and frequency problem. Women come to doctors with a problem which when not actually caused by their sexual activities has often interfered with them. Patients have often left a consultation with a general practitioner having learned that sex made them ill but without any ideas about how to cope with this. Doctors in the past have been too concerned about urine tests, kidney X-rays and even cystoscopies to notice such things. Treatment was seen largely as a prescription for a long course of antibiotics. Self-help groups have forced us to listen with a little more sympathy to the problems that people have; no general practitioner should ignore them.

GUIDELINES FOR THE GENERAL PRACTITIONER

The concept of significant bacteriuria (the Kass criterion of $10^8 \, cfu \, l^{-1}$) tells us that bacteria are multiplying in bladder urine which is a necessary prerequisite for the development of acute pyelonephritis. This information may not always be necessary or even helpful to the general practioner in determining the management and prognosis of individual cases of UTI in his practice.

Development of infection within the urinary tract is probably a continuous process. A diagnosis might be made at any stage. Any end-point must be arbitrary as must be any decision about antibacterial therapy. The need for urine bacteriology varies, then, according to the type of problem encountered and the type of information needed for management and prognosis. It also varies with the age and gender of the patient.

Women

Women with infrequent attacks of the dysuria and frequency syndrome may or may not have significant bacteriuria, but they are not at risk of renal scarring and kidney failure. Nor is their problem a particularly troublesome one. Is it always necessary to determine the presence or absence of significant bacteriuria either before or after treatment particularly if the cost of investigation outweighs the cost of treatment? Therapeutic intervention is hardly a serious matter, especially in view of the trend towards shorter courses, and symptomatic evidence of recovery would seem to be all that is necessary in most women who have infrequent attacks. Women with frequent attacks or severe constitutional symptoms however should have their urines examined bacteriologically from time to time in order to determine the pattern of attacks. Are cultures always negative or are some attacks accompanied by significant bacteriuria? What is the sensitivity pattern? Such women can be given a supply of dipslides which can be dropped in at the surgery before commencing treatment. Our overall aim must be to define the problem(s) accurately enough to prepare an acceptable management plan.

Many women with acute dysuria and frequency (perhaps one-third of all women during a 12-month period) are presenting with their very first attack which may reflect sexual activity and may be associated with feelings of guilt and anxiety about a pregnancy. They need an opportunity to talk about this as Thomas O'Dowd emphasizes in Chapter 2. Are MSUs and a physical examination really necessary in this group and in the many women with infrequent attacks and few constitutional symptoms? Women with frequent attacks do need careful assessment if only for reassurance purposes. Similarly how helpful are hospital diagnosis and management criteria when we come to make a decision about drug therapy?

The 'sore' urethra

Is there an analogy between the dysuria and frequency syndrome and sore throats? We know that most throat infections are viral in aetiology yet we do not swab all throats. We use clinical criteria to determine whether or not we will prescribe penicillin recognizing that bacteriological investigation is not particularly helpful. We may give aspirin to some streptococcal throats, but it hardly matters because most patients will get better anyway and complications are unlikely; if penicillin is given to some viral throats there is no real harm done.

We know that half the women with symptoms suggesting UTI will have significant bacteriuria and if we treat all those with symptoms some women may be given unnecessary treatment. Then again, many women with symptoms and significant bacteriuria will get better without antibacterial therapy. Is it unreasonable to give short courses of antibacterial treatment to all who have moderately severe symptoms? Whether or not we prescribe antibiotics the real challenge (as Thomas O'Dowd points out) is to identify patient concerns and expectations and look for factors that are relevant to pathogenesis. Women with mild symptoms can be given analgesics and encouraged to further the activity of their own natural defence mechanisms by drinking plenty of fluids.

Children

In contrast to women, UTI in children requires a different diagnostic and management approach, particularly for infants and pre-school children because of the possibility of renal scarring. It is necessary to identify children at risk which is difficult when symptoms and signs are vague and when typical symptoms do not necessarily denote infection. Bacteriological diagnosis is necessary if the right children are to be referred to hospital for further investigation as Robert Postlethwaite demonstrates so clearly in Chapter 4.

Men

Patrick Smith points out in Chapter 3 that men with pyelonephritis are ill, may not have significant bacteriuria, are usually in obvious need of hospital admission and always require a post treatment IVP.

Because of the proximity of the bladder, the prostate and the epididymis infection may on occasion involve all three. We must pay attention to the problem of chronic prostatitis which is compared with the 'urethral syndrome' in women, because of the difficulty in identifying pathogenic organisms and management problems.

The Elderly

As with young children perhaps the most important thing about infection in the elderly is to be aware that it may present only vague symptoms as Professor Brocklehurst and Dr Choudhury recommend. It is after all extremely common. He emphasizes the value of a 'trial of treatment'. If symptoms improve then infection is worth treating when it re-occurs.

References

1 Wulff, H. R. (1976). *Rational Diagnosis and Treatment*. (London: Blackwell Scientific Publications)

2 Kincaid-Smith, P. and Fairley, K. F. (1967). Diagnosis of urinary tract infection. *Hospital Med.* 993–998
3 Baird Parker, A. C. (1963). A classification of micrococci and staphylococci based on physiological and biochemical tests. *J. Gen. Microbiol.,* **30,** 409
4 Brooks, D. and Maudar, J. A. (1972). Urethral Syndrome in women and its diagnosis in general practice. *Lancet,* **2,** 893–898
5 Maskell, R. (1986). Are fastidious organisms an important cause of dysuria and frequency? In Asscher, A. W. and Brumfitt, W. (eds.) *Microbial Disease in Nephrology* (Chichester: John Wiley and Sons)
5 Numazaki, Y., Kumasaka, T., Yana, N. *et al.* (1973). *N. Engl. J. Med.,* **289,** 344
7 Kaye, D. (1975). Host defence mechanisms in the urinary tract. *Urol. Clin. N. Am.,* **2,** 407–422
8 Rovsing (1897) Quoted by Scholl, A. J. (1926). Cohabitation colon bacillary urinary tract infection. *J. Am. Med. Assoc.,* **87,** 1974
9 Moore, T. and Hira, N. A. (1965). The role of the female urethra in infections of the urinary tract. *Br. J. Urol.,* 37–25
10 Thomson, H. (1879). Remarks on the production of cystitis by contagion through the use of instruments. *Br. Med. J.,* **1,** 694
11 Kass, E. H. (1956). Asymptomatic infection of the urinary tract. *Trans. Assoc. Am. Phys.* **69,** 56
12 Kindall, L. and Nickells, T. T. (1949). Allergy of the pelvic urinary tract in the female. A preliminary report. *J. Urol.,* **61,** 222
13 Griffiths, L. C. and Kalton, G. (1972). Urinary Infection and symptoms of dysuria in women aged 54–64: their relevance to similar findings in the elderly. *Age Ageing,* **1,** 41–47
14 Tapsall, J. W., Bell, J. M., Taylor, P. C. and Smith, D. D. (1975). Relevance of significant bacteriuria to aetiology and diagnosis of urinary tract infection. *Lancet,* **2,** 537–639
15 Brumfitt, W., Smith, G. W. and Hamilton-Miller, J. M. T. (1986). Management of recurrent urinary tract infection. The place of a urinary infection clinic. In Asscher, A. W. and Brumfitt, W. (eds.) *Microbial Diseases in Nephrology,* p. 291. (Chichester: John Wiley and Sons)
16 Meers, P. D. (ed.) (1978). *The Bacteriological Examination of Urine.* Public Health Laboratory. Monograph Series No. 10. (London: HMSO)
17 Kass, E. H., Miall, W. E., Stuart, K. L. and Rosner, B. (1975). Epidemiologic aspects of infections of the urinary tract. In Kass, E. H. and Brumfitt, W. (eds) *Infections of the Urinary Tract.* (University of Chicago Press)

2

WOMEN WITH URINARY SYMPTOMS

T. C. O'DOWD

GENERAL CONSIDERATIONS

The size of the problem

One woman in five will experience lower urinary tract symptoms in a year yet only ten per cent will consult their doctor about these symptoms[1]. In only a small proportion of consulters and non-consulters will the symptoms indicate significant, serious illness (Figure 2.1). It is estimated that 50 per cent of women will experience a urinary tract infection (UTI) in their lifetimes and 50 per cent of these will relapse within a year. Two per cent of consultations in general practice are for urinary tract symptoms and UTI is said to be the commonest adult condition for which doctors prescribe an antibiotic[2].

A puzzle

However, the problem becomes even more intriguing when we realise that asymptomatic or covert bacteriuria (ASB) is the

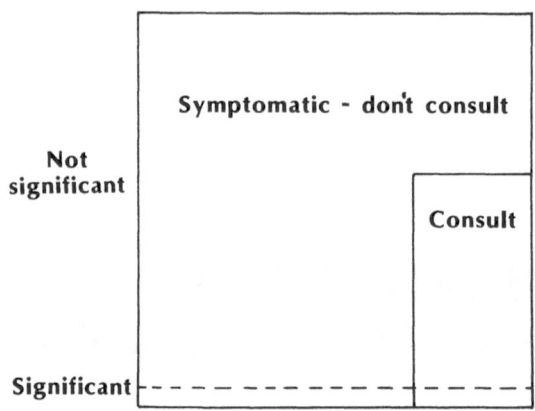

Figure 2.1 Urinary symptoms in women seen and not seen by doctors

commonest infection of the lower urinary tract. Such women have 10^5 or more organisms per ml of urine, which are only detected as part of a health screening programme. Five per cent of women between 16 and 65 years have ASB and 1 per cent undergo spontaneous remission per annum[3]. Why one group of women with 10^5 organisms per ml of urine should be completely asymptomatic whilst another group with the self-same infection have frequency and dysuria is surely one of the great puzzles of medicine.

The prescribing trap

When a woman with 'cystitis' or 'trouble with the waterworks' consults her doctor, quite often both fall into the trap of assuming they are dealing with a UTI. The general practitioner usually responds with an antibiotic and occasionally with an MSU bottle. However such symptoms may signify a host of

Table 2.1 Classification of urinary symptoms in women

(i) UTI: non-pregnant (young and old)
pregnant
(ii) Irritable urethral syndrome
(iii) Sexually transmissible diseases
(iv) Vaginitis: infective
senile
allergic

other conditions (Table 2.1). Of the women presenting with lower urinary tract symptoms only 50 per cent will have demonstrable infection to account for their complaints[4]. This group of women with UTI are divided into two groups for further consideration: non-pregnant and pregnant, because of differences in the possible consequences of infection.

NON-PREGNANT UTI

The non-pregnant woman with UTI will usually have *E. coli*, or far less commonly *Proteus sp.* or *staphylococcus*, to account for her symptoms. The consequences of a UTI for a non-pregnant woman are certainly not life-threatening. However 50 per cent will relapse within a year and many are sadly assigned to recurrent UTI and feeling systemically unwell. Such a pattern is not confined to young sexually active women. The elderly are particularly prone to recurrent UTI because of the associated structural changes that occur in the genito-urinary tract with ageing. Symptoms of systemic unwellness may predominate in the elderly, while frequency and dysuria predominate in the younger woman with UTI.

The first UTI

Patients with recurrent UTI often get a bad deal from doctors. A woman with her first UTI deserves counselling about

hygiene, sexual technique and prevention. The general practitioner (GP) may be tempted to treat each subsequent episode
as an event unconnected with the misery of past infections and
poorly predictive of the misery yet to come. Patients with gall
bladder disease and gout are advised about aggravating factors
and it is implied that they may have further trouble in the
future. Doctors develop a strategy in collaboration with such
patients because they see the condition in terms of chronicity;
recurrence implies episodic casualty-type medicine. It would
be helpful if we were to see a first UTI in these terms, as a
condition which may become chronic in a group of sexually
active women and elderly women.

Predisposing factors (Table 2.2)

Anatomical

The shortness of the female urethra permits easy access of gut
bacteria to the bladder. This process is triggered in young

Table 2.2   Factors predisposing to UTI in women

(i) Short urethra	(iii) Urinary pH and osmolality
(ii) Sexual intercourse:	(iv) Structural changes:
honeymoon	prolapse
holiday	post surgery
promiscuity	advancing years
	catheterisation

women by sexual intercourse. Indeed the shrewd doctor seeing
an adolescent complaining of lower urinary symptoms would
be wise to tactfully pursue the need for contraception. Further
advice may also be offered. If women empty their bladders
after intercourse this helps to flush out any organisms that
may have ascended during intercourse. Indeed French women
consider their British counterparts naive and unhygienic in not
douching as they do at the ever-present bidet in the bedroom

or toilet. Perfumed douches can of course cause allergic vaginitis and possible urethritis and are best avoided. In partners using barrier contraceptives allergy may develop to the spermicidal gel or cream or less commonly to the rubber used; a change of spermicide or diaphragm brand may help.

The urine

The PH and osmolality of female urine are often more suitable for bacterial growth than are those of male urine. In a classic experiment Asscher et al.[5] demonstrated that E. coli have great difficulty in growing in dilute urine and in urine with a pH greater than 7.5. This is the basis for advising women to drink plenty and to add bicarbonate of soda or mist. potassium citrate to a drink three or four times a day. Antiseptics like Mandelamine have been shown to be effective in controlling UTI[6].

Gentler remedies

Table 2.3 lists advice and remedies that will help the patient with chronic UTI. However patients and doctors who have become used to antibiotics may be resistant to suggestions that

Table 2.3   Home remedies for urinary symptoms

(i) Increased fluids	(v) Antiseptics:
(ii) Alkalinisation:	Mandelamine
bicarbonate of soda	(vi) Homeopathy:
Mist. Pot. Cit.	camphor
(iii) Rest	Arsenicum album
(iv) Avoid acidic fruits and	(vii) Diuretics:
juices	coffee
	DeWitts pills

they pursue older gentler remedies. They are reminded that while antibiotics kill off the organisms, the symptoms may persist after the organisms have gone. Indeed, in a study of antibiotic and placebo treatment of UTI, there was no difference in the duration of symptoms or recurrence rates between the two groups in the first year after treatment[7].

Homeopathic text books[8] demonstrate greater sophistication in history taking in the urinary tract than do conventional medical text books. We should keep an open mind; a number of women have become disenchanted with conventional medical treatment of urinary disorders[9]. The great strength of trying a new method of treatment may be that it makes us more interested in eliciting the case history and observing the outcome. We have, after all, often become quite cavalier in our simplistic faith in antibiotics.

A management strategy (Figure 2.2)

Nowadays we trust patients to measure their own blood glucose, adjust their anticoagulation treatment and check their intrauterine devices. It can hardly be considered revolutionary to allow women to initiate their own antibiotic treatment in chronic UTI if their symptoms have not responded to fluids and chosen remedies. An occasional MSU may be needed to check the organism present and the development of any

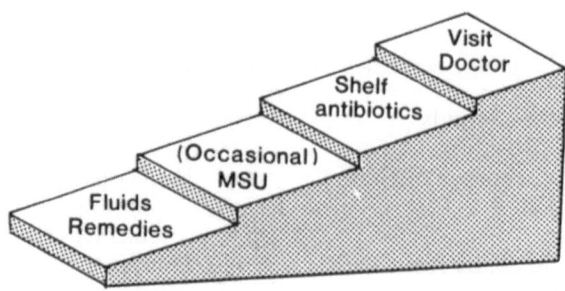

Figure 2.2   Chronic (recurrent) UTI: a management strategy

antibiotic resistance; the doctor need only be visited for repeat MSU bottles, laboratory forms and antibiotics for the bathroom-shelf. If the pattern of infection and symptomatology show any changes or resistance emerges then re-evaluation of the treatment is needed. Otherwise such patients can manage well on their own.

THE URETHRAL SYNDROME (abacterial cystitis)

In 1965 a group of New Zealand GPs coined the term 'urethral syndrome' (US) to describe the 50 per cent of their female patients with urinary symptoms but without demonstrable infection[4]. This syndrome has been welcomed as a challenge by clinicians and microbiologists looking for a microbiological cause. However, the populations studied suffer from selection bias, being referred patients, students or genito-urinary clinic patients.

Chlamydia trachomatis is the organism most commonly associated with the urethral syndrome in sexually active promiscuous populations. A low incidence of *Chlamydia* has been found in routine family planning clinics[10] and amongst hospital staff volunteers[11]. Two general practice studies of symptomatic women failed to isolate any *Chlamydia*[12, 13] while one inner city study of women with genito-urinary and vaginal problems found *Chlamydia* in 8 per cent of cases[14]. Most of these *Chlamydia*-positive studies are really describing chlamydial cervicitis, urethritis or vaginitis and not the urethral syndrome. Nonetheless in a woman with persistent painful symptoms and a promiscuous lifestyle the clinician would be wise to consider *Chlamydia*. It is also worth remembering that *Chlamydia* has a higher isolation rate in women who already have *Trichomonas vaginale* and gonorrhoea.

Recent general practice studies on the urethral syndrome showed that it was a short self-limiting illness and that dysuria was much less in the urethral syndrome than in conventional UTI[12, 15]. In addition it has been shown that doctors were able to predict in advance of the MSU which women had UTI and which had US on the basis of the amount of dysuria and the psychological make-up of the patient[15]. Those with US were more likely to suffer anxiety symptoms than UTI controls. In a further follow-up study, these women described themselves as less healthy than asymptomatic controls and were more likely to mention health problems affecting their sex lives[15, 17, 18]. Table 2.4 gives a summary of the differences between UTI and urethral syndrome.

Table 2.4 Markers distinguishing irritable urethral syndrome (IUS) from urinary tract infection (UTI)

Marker	IUS	UTI
Frequency	+	+
Dysuria	−	+
Pus cells	Scanty	> 5/HPF
Consultation rate	High	Average
Anxiety symptoms	Many	Few
Contraception	Sterilised	Various
Relationship problems	Many	Few
Feel healthy	No	Yes

HPF = High power field

Irritable urethral syndrome

Urethral syndrome is a term that has not been entirely accept-able to our specialist colleagues[19]. The Medical Research Bac-teriuria Committee (1979) has recommended that it should be called the 'frequency and dysuria syndrome'. However this title does not recognize the fact that many of these women do not have dysuria. Indeed the syndrome has more in common with the irritable bowel syndrome than it has with UTI[13]. Both conditions are commoner in women who perceive themselves as unhealthy and are high demand and anxious. Both con-ditions commonly coexist in the same patient and they are a great drain on the GP's time and emotion. Perhaps if we thought of the condition as the irritable urethral syndrome these women might be given less cursory treatment.

Management

Asking doctors to pursue a psychosocial management plan for a condition that may have an organic basis causes clinical insecurity. Indeed the patient herself may not accept a psychosocial model for her complaint; one has only to read Angela Kilmartin's book *Understanding Cystitis*[9] – anger and frustration are glinting through its pages. Nonetheless we do sit down with patients with the irritable bowel syndrome and *negotiate* a psychosomatic aspect to the condition. The trouble with urethral syndrome is that it is a diagnosis by default as it is rarely recorded in patients' notes. The diagnosis may be missed because of reflex prescription of an antibiotic or it may pass through our fingers as the receptionist tells the patient over the phone that 'your water test was perfectly alright – nothing to worry about'. This management does not solve the problem, for such women reappear with the IUS for consultation three to four times a year[20].

It has to be admitted that there is no magic management plan for the irritable urethral syndrome. It is in the company of a host of other conditions that doctors diagnose but can do very little about. Perhaps the kindest thing that can be done for a woman with IUS is to resist the temptation to refer. Such women have been subjected to barbaric treatments like urethrotomy, urethral dilatation and steroid injections into the urethra and occasional specialists may still be tempted to try such methods more out of frustration than because of any therapeutic rationale.

VAGINITIS AND URINARY SYMPTOMS

About 5 per cent of women with vaginitis will present to their doctor with lower urinary tract symptoms[6]. Good history taking should however enable the doctor to pinpoint them. If the dysuria persists after micturition is finished vaginitis should be considered. Other symptoms of vaginitis should also be sought: intercourse-related discomfort, discharge and pruritus. Prescribing an antibiotic to such women may only make the vaginitis worse since this may induce thrush. It is only worthwhile doing a vaginal examination on women with lower urinary tract symptoms where the history also suggests a vaginitis or vaginal prolapse.

Diagnostic aids

Urinoscopy

Many women bring a urine sample to back up their claim that they have 'cystitis'. It is well worthwhile inspecting the urine under good light (urinoscopy). Clear urine is nearly always bacteriologically negative while a woman with vaginitis may have streaks of mucus floating around in the sample. Crystals lend a cloudy appearance to urine which may be misinterpreted as pyuria. Placing a drop of uncentrifuged urine on a glass slide under a microscope will quickly distinguish crystals from pus cells.

Microscopy

Microscopy has fallen out of favour with doctors. The decline began when ward side-rooms got rid of their microscopes and junior doctors and medical students lost the opportunity of learning how useful they could be. Many practices have microscopes lying in cupboards begging to be used. They are discovered every now and then during a spring clean and a 'small ad' is promptly placed in the weekly medical newspapers. The interested doctor may take advantage of this and get started for a relatively modest outlay; a good instruction book on microscopy is Sister Laurine Graaff's *Handbook of Routine Urinalysis*[21].

FURTHER STEPS TO TAKE

Check MSU

There is a counsel of perfection that says that a check MSU should be performed after treating a UTI but in practice this is rarely done. Indeed, it is unnecessary in uncomplicated UTI because of the effectiveness of antibiotics; the UTI will clear on its own eventually and in the case of a relapse the MSU will only corroborate the patient's diagnosis anyway.

When to refer

The referral threshold for women with urinary symptoms varies with the knowledge, skills and facilities that the individual general practitioner can rely upon. There is a lot of negotiation to be done with a woman who develops chronic infection or the irritable urethral syndrome. There is much clinical uncertainty to be tolerated by doctor and patient whilst negotiation goes on. In view of past treatments of women with the IUS, the general practitioner may have to play a protective role in preventing more invasive specialist procedures. The GP who clearly states his/her objective in the referral letter to a carefully chosen consultant is exercising this protective role. Some guidelines for referral are shown in Table 2.5.

Table 2.5   Guidelines for referral of women with lower urinary tract problems

---

(i)   Possible sexually transmissible cause
(ii)   Infections with rarer organisms, e.g., *Pseudomonas*
(iii)   Persistant pyuria despite treatment
(iv)   History of renal stones

SEXUALLY TRANSMITTED DISEASES

It is surprising how rarely patients consult their GP about sexually transmitted diseases (STD). Patients who suspect that their symptoms may be due to STD select the genito-urinary clinic instead of the GP. This is for a variety of reasons ranging from the wish to be anonymous to the knowledge that such

Table 2.6 Sexually transmitted diseases: at risk groups

(i)   Promiscuity (either partner)
(ii) Some ethnic groups
(iii) Teenagers
(iv) Low IQ
(v)   Homo-/bisexual

clinics are better equipped to deal with investigation and follow-up. Up to 25 per cent of attendances at STD clinics are for reassurance alone[22]. However the GP may still see women with urinary problems from STD. Certain groups of women are at risk (Table 2.6), some by default rather than by intent. Some of these patients may not want referral to an STD clinic and if the doctor is happy that contact tracing would be fruitless then diagnosis must be undertaken.

Towards a diagnosis of STD

It is important to remember that there may be more than one offending venereal organism causing the symptoms. The GP is often baffled by the array of swabs and bottles needed for the diagnosis of STD. Table 2.7 gives a summary of the required investigation. Five cotton wool swabs are needed. A high vaginal swab of any discharge is performed for *Candida* and *Gardnerella* and another for *Trichomonas*. The cervix should be swabbed for chlamydia and *Gonococcus* while any herpetic lesions present should also be swabbed for herpes

Table 2.7 Investigation for the woman with urinary symptoms of STD origin

Organism	Swab	Medium	Storage
Chlamydia	Cervix/urethra	Chlamydia Transport Microtrack	4°C (refrigerator)
Herpes	Lesions	Virus Transport	4°C
Trichomonas	Discharge (HVS)	Trichomonas Growth	Room temperature
Candida	Discharge/ plaques	Stuarts	Room temperature
Gardnerella	Discharge (HVS)	Stuarts	Room temperature
Gonococcus	Cervix/urethra	Stuarts	Body temperature

HVS = high vaginal swab

labialis. Without doubt *Gonococcus* is the most fragile of the venereal organisms and liable to die if stored for long. If doctor and patient go to the trouble of doing so many swabs then the patient should be prepared to transport them immediately to the local laboratory. It is worth mentioning that many women who suspect they are going to have a vaginal examination will have a bath beforehand, thus washing away a lot of discharge which can make swabbing more difficult.

UTI IN PREGNANCY

Infection of the urine in pregnancy increases the stakes dramatically. The incidence of ASB in pregnancy is between 4 and 7 per cent – which is similar to that of the non-pregnant population. However one third of women with ASB in pregnancy will go on to develop pyelonephritis if not treated. Pyelonephritis predisposes to prematurity and neonatal death. Thus screening for ASB at the first antenatal visit is an extremely worthwhile exercise that is usually carried out at the booking appointment. However, the screening MSU and its result are seldom recorded for the GP despite the use of a shared care card. Some hospitals even send antibiotics through the post to those women who have ASB which surely must count as a dangerous activity.

Symptomatic lower urinary tract infection in pregnancy should be managed in a similar fashion to that of the non-pregnant woman with due consideration of the safety of the antibiotic chosen. Interestingly the irritable urethral syndrome does not seem to occur in pregnancy.

A post partum IVP

It may come as a surprise to many GPs to hear that it is widely recommended that a woman with ASB should have an intravenous pyelogram (IVP) 3 to 6 months after the birth of the baby. If this policy is actually being fully implemented it means that 37 500 young women are having IVPs in Britain annually or that each District General Hospital is doing over three IVPs per week[23]. The existence of this policy reflects research done in the 1960s where, in one study in Melbourne[24], 50 per cent of women with ASB were shown to have abnormal IVPs. By 1968, Gower et al.[25], in London, diagnosed only 18 per cent of women with ASB as having abnormal IVPs. In the Melbourne study, the IVP was performed 6 weeks after delivery, before the hormonal effects on the ureters had subsided, and it may be that the population was prone to renal damage from habitual phenacetin ingestion (this was widespread in Australia in the 1960s). The London study was more selective in what were considered to be renal abnormalities. The abnormalities were divided into major and minor, though a classification of what was and was not amenable to treatment would have cleared the air much more. Eight per cent of women were considered to have major renal abnormalities though three quarters of these had renal scarring from childhood pyelonephritis. A second Australian study[26] in 1972 replicated the London findings and found that 60 per cent of those with major renal abnormalities had had a past history of renal disease. The authors were more forthright in their conclusions: most of the major renal abnormalities they found could be expected to turn up when the clinical situation demanded investigation. Doing IVPs in all cases of bacteriuria is unwarranted and leads to many radiological abnormalities of uncertain significance being found.

An IVP post pyelonephritis?

Pyelonephritis in pregnancy is much commoner in women with ASB in the third trimester because the ureters are dilated and the weight of the uterus on the ureters causes stasis and thus infection. This is widely accepted as a cause of pyelonephritis and seems very reasonable. Yet it is widely recommended that all such women should have an IVP. This seems to have arisen because of the link between ASB and pyelonephritis in pregnancy. The fears and assumptions about ASB were felt to be vindicated when the ascending bacteria had succeeded in roosting in the kidney. There is little evidence to support these fears and assumptions.

It must be remembered, however, that pyelitis of pregnancy was once the commonest complication of pregnancy, causing a maternal mortality of 3–4 per cent and a foetal loss from prematurity of 16–30 per cent at the start of the antibiotic era[27]. The memories of such mortality have dictated the way researchers of the 1960s interpret their findings. In the 1980s, however, obstetricians have not revised their policies despite antenatal screening, antibiotic therapy, regular antenatal care and healthier women. It would be worthwhile repeating those earlier studies now, with the added benefits of less invasive radiological techniques and more realistic interpretation of the findings.

Who should have an IVP then? (Table 2.8)

Pyelonephritis responds quickly to antibiotics. It would be prudent to do a post partum IVP on any patient with a slow or partial response to treatment. Women with a past history of renal disease seem to have a highly predictive marker of a major renal abnormality[25] and are worthy of investigation. Should the urine grow a rarer organism like *Pseudomonas* it is worth thinking of an obstructive cause. The case for doing an IVP in ASB of pregnancy also needs to be re-examined. Certainly an IVP should be considered for a patient developing a second infection with a different organism but a second infection with the same organism may merely be a relapse. A repeated post partum MSU for bacteriuria and albumen is sufficient.

Table 2.8 Proposed indications for a post partum IVP

(i) Pyelonephritis:	slow/partial response to treatment
	past history of pyelonephritis
	isolation of rarer organism
(ii) ASB/UTI:	second infection: different organism

Treatment of UTI in women

Over the last 10 years antibiotic treatment of UTI has become of shorter and shorter duration. Yet many doctors continue

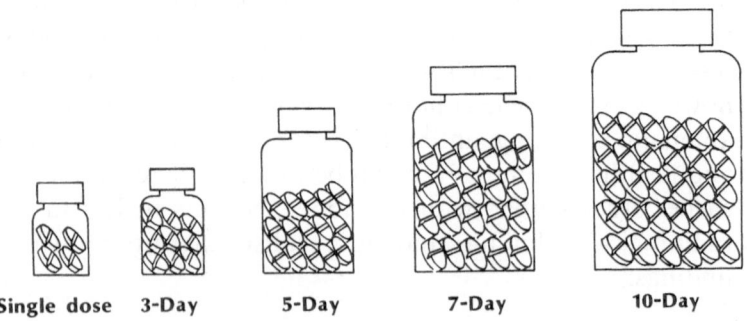

Single dose   3-Day   5-Day   7-Day   10-Day

Figure 2.3   Uncomplicated UTI: how long to treat?

to use a wide range in the length of antibiotic courses they give their patients (Figure 2.3). Without doubt we have been overtreating uncomplicated UTI in the past.

How long should treatment be?

The choice has really come down to a single dose or a 3-day treatment. There is ample evidence to show that 10-day treatment is no better than 8-day treatment with respect to eradication of organisms, relief of symptoms and prevention of reinfection[28]. It is worth mentioning again that relief of symptoms takes longer than eradication of organisms and, indeed, that clearance of symptoms may not mean eradication of organisms.

Single doses of 2 g of sulfadoxine[29], 3 g of amoxycillin[30] and 2.88 g of co-trimoxazole[31] have all been tried against conventional treatment and found to be successful. The striking feature of the single dose regimes used is the size of the dose. Three grams of amoxycillin is equivalent to four days treatment with 250 mg capsules t.i.d.

More recently 1 g of amoxycillin has been found to be effective[32] and four tablets of trimethoprim (400 mg) or four tablets of co-trimoxazole[33] are as effective as the conventional seven days treatment.

The advantages of short or single dose therapy are fewer side effects and better compliance. These monetarist times have led to speculation that a saving of 1 million pounds per year could be made by switching from seven day to single dose treatment of UTI[33].

Chronic UTI

'Low dose' prophylaxis of UTI in children has been very successful in preventing renal damage[34] and in preventing reinfection[35]. When counselling and radiological investigations do not reveal a cause and the patient gets frequent infection, then low dose prophylaxis of one antibiotic tablet a day may help. However the patient herself may prefer the strategy (Figure 2.2) of a few short courses of antibiotic throughout the years when she is symptomatic.

Post-coital prophylaxis

A few women can pinpoint the onset of their infection to the act of sexual intercourse. In those women in whom bladder emptying immediately afterwards is not effective a single antibiotic tablet post-coitally may prevent the misery of yet another infection.

PRACTICAL POINTS

● Urinary infection is common in women. Up to one half of all women experience infection at some time in their lives and of these one half relapse within a year. Why some have symptoms and some do not is one of medicine's great puzzles. Indeed we also remain uncertain why only half of those with symptoms have bacteriuria.

● A first infection may herald a chronic illness in some women. Women presenting with a first infection may benefit from counselling (contraception, sexual technique, hygiene, prevention).

● Advice such as emptying the bladder after sexual intercourse and douching in a bidet may be helpful to some women with recurrent symptoms as may drinking plenty of fluids, alkalinisation of the urine, rest and avoiding acidic fruits and juices.

● Women with chronic symptoms can be trusted to initiate their own antibiotic therapy.

● There are some women with chronic symptoms who never have significant bacteriuria. It is helpful to regard them as having an irritable urethra syndrome. This can be compared with the irritable bowel syndrome in that addressing psycho-social factors may be a helpful management approach.

● Post-treatment MSUs are unnecessary in uncomplicated infections.

● Too many women with recurrent symptoms have been referred to consultant colleagues in previous years. Guide-lines for referral include a possible sexually transmissible cause, infection with a rare organism, persistant pyuria and a history of renal stones.

● Screening is worthwhile in pregnant women. One-third of patients with covert bacteriuria go on to develop pyelone-phritis if not treated. Pyelonephritis predisposes to prema-turity and neonatal death as well as being a particularly distressing illness.

● A postpartum IVP after pyelonephritis in pregnancy is worthwhile in any patient with a slow or partial response to treatment, in women with a past history of renal disease, and when there is a rare organism responsible for the infection. When bacteriuria is asymptomatic a second infection with a different organism merits a post partum IVP.

● The choice for treatment of UTI in women has come down to single dose or 3-day treatment. Sulfadoxine (2 g), amoxy-cillin (3 g), and co-trimoxazole (2.88 g) have all been re-commended as single doses.

● Prophylactic therapy with one antibiotic tablet a day is of great help to women with troublesome recurrent symptoms. An alternative is to provide the patient with enough tablets to allow early treatment of frequently occurring attacks. Post coital prophylaxis is of value in some women.

References

1. Waters, W. E. (1969). Prevalence of symptoms of urinary tract infection in women. *Br. J. Preventive Soc Med.*, **23**, 263–266

2. Brooks, D. and Mallick, N. (1982). Infections of the urine and urinary tract. In *Renal Medicine and Urology*. p. 56. (Edinburgh: Churchill Livingstone)

3. Asscher, A. W. (1980). *The Challenge of Urinary Tract Infections*. (London: Academic Press)

4. Gallagher, D. J. A., Montgomerie, J. Z. and North, J. D. K. (1965). Acute infections of the urinary tract and the urethral syndrome in general practice. *Br. Med. J.*, **1**, 622–626

5. Asscher, A. W., Sussman, M., Waters, W. E. *et al.* (1966). Urine as a medium for bacterial growth. *Lancet*, **2**, 1037–1039

6. Rosenheim, M. L. (1935). Mandelic acid in the treatment of urinary infections. *Lancet*, **1** 1032–1037

7. Mabeck, C. E. (1972). Treatment of uncomplicated urinary tract infections in non-pregnant women. *Postgrad. Med. J.*, **48**, 69–75

8. Pratt, N. (1985). *Homeopathic Prescribing*. (Beaconsfield, Bucks: Beaconsfield Publishers Ltd.)

9. Kilmartin, A. (1973). *Understanding Cystitis*. (London: Pan Books Ltd)

10. Hilton A. L., Richmond, S. J., Milne, J. D., Hindley, F. and Clarke S. K. R. (1974). *Chlamydia A* in the female genital tract. *Br. J. Vener. Dis.*, **50**, 1–9

11. Woolfitt, J. M. G. and Watt, L. (1979). Chlamydial infection of the urogenital tract in promiscuous and non-promiscuous women. *Br. J. Vener. Dis.*, **53**, 93–95

12. Burney, P., Marson, W. S., Evans, M. and Forsey, T. (1983). *Chlamydia trachomatis* and lower urinary tract symptoms among women in one general practice. *Br. Med. J.*, **286**, 1550–1552

13. O'Dowd, T. C., Ribeiro, C. D., Munro, J. A., West, R. R. and Howells C. H. L. (1984). The urethral syndrome – a self limiting illness. *Br. Med. J.*, **288**, 1349–1352

14. Southgate, L. J., Treharne, J. D. and Forsey, T. (1983). *Chlamydia trachomatis* and *Neisseria* gonorrhoeal infections in women attending inner city general practices. *Br. Med. J.* **287**, 1277–1280

15. O'Dowd, T. C., Smail, J. E. and West R. R. (1984). Clinical judgement in the management of frequency and dysuria in general practice. *Br. Med. J.* **288**, 1397–1349

16. O'Dowd, T. C. (1985). The irritable urethral syndrome: discussion. *J. R. Coll. Gen. Pract.*, **35**, 140–141

17. O'Dowd, T. C., Pill, R., Smail, J. E. and Davis, R. H. (1986). The irritable urethral syndrome: a follow up study in general practice. *Br. Med. J.*, **292**, 30–32

18. O'Dowd, T. C., West, R. R., Ribeiro, C. D., Smail, J. E. and Munro, J. A. (1986). The contribution of *Gardnerella vaginitis* to vaginitis in general practice. *Br. Med. J.*, **292**, 1640–1642

19. Report by members of the Medical Research Council Bacteriuria Committee. (1979). Recommended terminology of urinary tract infection. *Br. Med. J.*, **2**, 717–719

20. Brooks, D. (1978). A general practitioner's view of the laboratory examination of urine. In Meers, P. D. (ed.) *The Bacteriological Exam-*

ination of Urine: Report of a Workshop on Needs and Methods, pp. 39–44. *Public Health Laboratory Service.* (London: HMSO)

21. Graaff, L. (1982). *A Handbook of Routine Urinalysis.* (Philadelphia: J. B. Lippincott Company)

22. Adler, M. W. (1983). ABC of sexually transmitted diseases. A changing and growing problem. *Br. Med. J.,* **287,** 1279–1281

23. Fry, J., Brooks, D. and MColl, I. (1984). *NHS DATA Book.* (Lancaster: MTP Press)

24. Kincaid-Smith, P. and Bullen, M. (1965). Bacteriuria in pregnancy. *Lancet,* **1,** 395–399

25. Gower, P. E., Heswell, B., Sidaway, M. E. and De Wardener, H. E. (1968). Follow up of 164 patients with bacteriuria of pregnancy. *Lancet,* **1,** 990–994

26. Briedahl, P., Hurst, P. E., Martin, J. S. and Vivian, A. B. (1972). The post partum investigation of pregnancy bacteriuria. *Med. J. Aust.,* **2,** 1174–1177

27. Hurley, R. (1984). Fewer and infectious diseases. In de Swiet, M. (ed.) *Medical Disorders in Obstetric Practice,* pp. 483–497. (London: Blackwell Scientific Publications)

28. Charlton, C. A. C. (1980). Ultra-short treatment of urinary tract infection. In Asscher, A. W. (ed.) *The Management of Urinary Tract Infection.* pp. 81–84. (Oxford: The Medicine Publishing Foundation)

29. Gruneberg, R. N. and Bramfitt, W. (1967). Single dose treatment of acute UTIs. *Br. Med. J.,* **iii,** 649–651

30. Bailey, R. R. and Abbott, G. D. (1977). Treatment of urinary tract infections with a single dose of Amoxycillin. *Nephrology,* **18,** 316

31. Bailey, R. R. and Abbott, G. D. (1978). Treatment of urinary tract infections with a single dose of Trimethoprim Sulfamethoxazole. *Can. Med. Assoc. J.,* **118,** 551–552

32. Anderson, J. D., Aird, M. Y., Johnson, A. M. *et al.* (1979). The use of 1 g dose of Amoxycillin for the treatment of urinary tract infections. *J. Antimicrob. Chemother.,* **5,** 481–483

33. Jones, R. H. (1983). Single dose and seven day trimethaprim and co-trimoxazole in the treatment of urinary tract infection. *J. R. Coll. Gen. Pract.,* **33,** 585–589

34. Smellie, J. M. and Normand, I. C. S. (1968). Experience of follow up of children with urinary tract infection. In O'Grady, F. W. and Brumfitt, W. (eds.) *Urinary Tract Infection.* (Oxford: Oxford University Press)

35. Smellie, J. M., Katz, G. and Gruneberg, R. N. (1978). Controlled trial of prophylactic treatment in childhood urinary tract infection. *Lancet,* **2,** 175–178

3

MEN WITH URINARY TRACT INFECTION

P. SMITH

INTRODUCTION

The male urinary tract, unlike its female counterpart, is in some measures protected from infection due to the presence of an extended urethral opening well away from the bacterial population of the perineum and peri-anal areas. However this relative security is counterbalanced by a much greater involvement of the male urinary tract with its adjoining genital tract (Figure 3.1). This association, especially as it relates to the prostate gland and posterior urethra, is a major contributor to the incidence of urinary infection in the male.

There is also a more formal clinical demarcation into upper and lower urinary tract infections in the male than in the female. Upper urinary tract infections are almost always due to discrete sepsis producing localized pyelonephritis. Lower urinary tract infections remain generally confined to the bladder or the adjoining genital areas of prostate, vas and epididymis. This anatomical differentiation of male urinary tract infection is reflected in a distinct pattern of pathogenesis and, due to the absence of a vaginal 'sump'[1], a different pattern

55

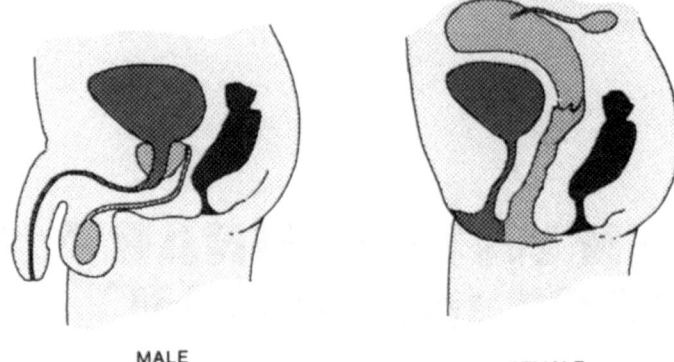

MALE

FEMALE

Figure 3.1   Differing associations of urinary and genital tracts in male and female

of infecting organisms. There are correspondingly different approaches to the treatment of infection in the male: long-term chemotherapy may be preferred in contrast to attempts to improve urethral drainage.

For practical purposes it is possible to divide infections of the male urinary tract into three different groups.

(1) Infection confined to the upper urinary tract: pyelo-nephritis.

(2) Infection involving the bladder: 'cystitis'.

(3) Infection arising primarily in the genital tract: loosely defined as prostatitis.

INFECTIONS OF THE UPPER URINARY TRACT – PYELONEPHRITIS

Infections of the renal parenchyma and pelvis are uncommon in the male. The majority of cases where they arise are related solely to upper tract disease and, unlike the female, are seldom associated with lower urinary tract problems. The causes of

AETIOLOGY OF PYELONEPHRITIS

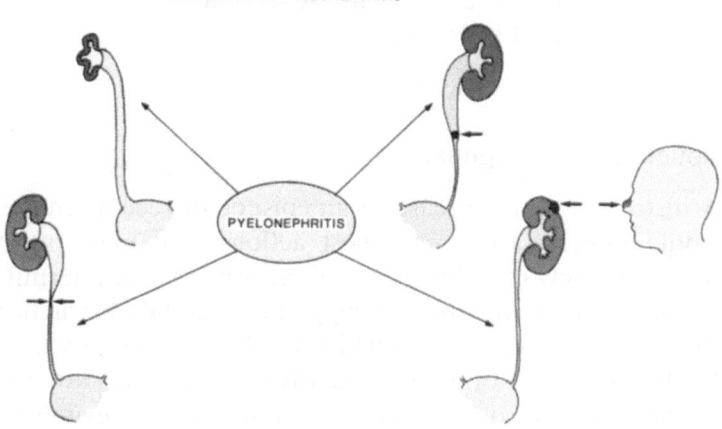

Figure 3.2 Aetiology of pyelonephritis in the male

adult male pyelonephritis are almost always due to stasis (Figure 3.2). The commonest presentation of such stasis is stone disease with a combination of obstruction and secondary infection. More rarely such obstruction is found in association with congenital hydronephrosis due to pelvi-ureteric junction obstruction or hydronephrosis due to congenital obstructions of the ureter lower down. Rarely, metastatic infection, usually a staphylococcus from a skin infection, may cause an initial acute focal pyelonephritis with the subsequent formation of a renal carbuncle. Pyelonephritis due to vesico-ureteric reflux, though common in children and occasionally seen in young adult women, is virtually non-existent in men.

Men with pyelonephritis are ill. This is the first and most important feature of diagnosis. They complain of malaise and generally of loin pain. They may have frequency and dysuria but this is not an inevitable feature of pyelonephritis in men since the infected urine is often trapped in the kidney due to obstruction and cannot therefore reach the bladder to present as a 'cystitis'. Similarly, unlike the female where the lower urinary tract is the usual source of upper tract infection, initial 'cystitis' symptoms are rare in the male as his pyelonephritis is primarily renal in origin.

Aetiology and diagnosis

A history of stone disease or an episode of recent renal colic would indicate the commonest aetiology of male pyelone-phritis, namely calculus obstruction. A history of intermittent long-standing loin pain may suggest congenital obstruction of the renal pelvis or a ureter which has been previously aseptic. In the rare event of a subsequently proven metastatic pyelo-nephritis a story of skin infection some weeks previously can sometimes be obtained. This type of renal infection is rare however and the skin sepsis is often quite remote from the actual pyelonephritis – making it a retrospective comment in most histories. Finally, a previous history of contralateral renal disease or even nephrectomy makes management of a pyelonephritis in a solitary kidney even more exacting.

As with all physical examination of the urinary tract, physi-cal signs of pyelonephritis are few. However men with pyelone-phritis, it is worth re-emphasizing, are often very ill. A high temperature is usually present and loin tenderness is marked. It is important to test the urine but, as mentioned above, the results can be misleading in that the urinary sepsis is often trapped behind an obstruction so that pyuria and organisms will fail to show on routine urinalysis of bladder urine. A normal MSU therefore (and this is important in clinical prac-tice) does not negate a diagnosis of pyelonephritis.

The diagnosis of male pyelonephritis may therefore be made on history and examination alone.

Management

The immediate treatment is rest, fluids and antibiotics. For most cases oral trimethoprim or ampicillin are sufficient and such antibiotic therapy is usually continued for 14 days. However a clinical response should be evident within the first few days. If this does not occur then additional therapy with parenteral cephalosporin or even aminoglycoside drugs is indicated.

Additional antibiotic therapy is usually preceded by hospital admission since the general illness of these men at this stage will make home care very difficult. In addition, when pyelonephritis does not respond immediately to oral therapy this may be an indication of mechanical obstruction such as stone. It is a matter of urgency that any obstruction be identified and released in order to bring any infection under control. Delay in diagnosis here can result in a pyonephrosis as well as pyelonephritis with kidney destruction following. Hospital admission is essential: intravenous pyelogram and ultrasound studies can be performed. If these show obstruction then relief by percutaneous nephrostomy or indwelling ureteric catheter (stent) are performed as an emergency. Once drainage is established antibiotic therapy becomes effective and subsequent formal surgery such as stone extraction or destruction can be performed at leisure.

All patients, whether requiring hospital admission or no, require close follow-up to clear up any underlying disease, especially obstruction, and to assess any long-term damage to kidney function. Even those responding to antibiotics require a follow-up intravenous pyelogram (IVP) to eliminate the possibility of any intermittent obstruction – the major predisposing cause in men. Urine culture is needed to confirm the elimination of urinary sepsis. These tests can be performed 2–4 weeks after the initial presentation and relief of clinical pyelonephritis. Patients who were admitted to hospital will have had these studies performed already. It cannot be stressed enough, however, how essential it is to prevent further episodes of pyelonephritis by permanently removing any upper urinary tract obstruction. It is clear therefore that all men must at some stage have an IVP following an episode of pyelonephritis and the sooner the better.

This condition of pyelonephritis in men is rare and the patients are usually so ill that virtually all merit hospital admission both for conservative treatment, investigation and, as is usually the case, surgical correction of any drainage impairment. Finally the rare incidence of renal carbuncle, while not requiring drainage, may occasionally need needle aspiration of the abscess – again an indication for hospital-based management.

INFECTIONS OF THE LOWER URINARY TRACT – 'CYSTITIS'

Urinary infection involving the bladder is not nearly as common in men as women. It is, however, just as miserable and debilitating a condition and requires prompt and effective management. Because of the protection given by the long male urethra, bladder infections are rarely due to ascending contaminants though, as will be seen below, this can occur in prostatitis. In most cases men develop 'cystitis' secondary to urinary stasis which in turn relates to obstruction. The commonest site of such obstruction is at the bladder outlet and the commonest cause is prostatic disease[1].

Symptomatology and differential diagnosis

The symptoms of 'cystitis' are classically the sudden onset of frequency and dysuria sometimes associated with haematuria. In some cases urgency and even urge incontinence may present at a later stage. The symptoms arise as a result of detrusor (bladder muscle) irritability and bladder and urethral mucosal sensitivity. There are usually, though to the patient often not in themselves worrying, additional symptoms of underlying prostatism with frequency and nocturia due to mechanical detrusor instability combined with hesitancy, poor stream and terminal dribbling due to dysfunction at the bladder neck.

These obstructive symptoms, of course, constitute the syndrome of prostatism itself.

Though this classic situation of obstruction, urinary stasis and secondary sepsis is usually clearly defined in men it is important to differentiate an equally important group of symptoms which can masquerade as cystitis. These can be loosely linked together as 'chronic cystitis'. In these men the story is of long-standing, unrelenting and progressive frequency and dysuria, often with haematuria and occasionally incontinence. These symptoms arise due to either an actual or a functional contracture of the bladder. The important feature is the chronic nature of the symptoms and the lack of any underlying obstructive disease. Such chronic cystitis is non-suppurative and can arise due to malignant cystitis caused by anaplastic or *in situ* bladder carcinoma or to interstitial 'cystitis' resulting from a curious and little understood degeneration of the bladder wall. Both these conditions are non-infective but their symptoms will often cause confusion in diagnosis at an early stage. Though uncommon they should be carefully considered in any men with longstanding 'cystitis' symptoms.

Routine physical examination of men with 'cystitis' is usually unrewarding. Unlike men with pyelonephritis, patients with cystitis are usually quite well in themselves. Bladder enlargement is very occasionally found but this is rare. Examination of the prostate is required only in order to identify the occasional case of malignant obstruction caused by a hard, irregular prostatic carcinoma. The size of the prostate itself is irrelevant to management, both in relation to cystitis and, indeed, to straightforward prostatism.

However, prostate hypertrophy (as a consequence of reduced voiding pressure and the inevitable pressure of a residual urine) may result in bacterial cystitis and transurethral prostatectomy may be necessary. Less than 10 per cent of men with primary bacterial cystitis ever require transurethral surgery.

Urine culture is mandatory in each case of diagnosis for

Table 3.1   The causes of sterile pyuria

  (i) Infection following chemotherapy
 (ii) Chronic pyelonephritis
(iii) Tuberculous disease of the urinary tract
(iv) Malignant infected cystitis, i.e., chronic *in situ* carcinoma

---

cystitis. Microscopy is most important for confirming the presence of infection as shown by pus cells. Other causes of sterile pyuria must not be forgotten; this is particularly important for patients with 'chronic cystitis' (see Table 3.1). Where there is doubt a urine cytology to identify malignant cells can readily be performed. Culture of the urine will identify any infecting organisms in routine cystitis cases. In men there is usually little difficulty in producing an absolute count of organisms to clinch the diagnosis since urethral contaminants, unlike the female, rarely present any problems.

Management

Treatment of urinary infection is by oral antibiotics: trimethoprim and Augmentin are most efficient. However the older generation of nitrofurantoin and nalidixic acid are just as effective. Rarely is it necessary to employ more complex drugs such as new generation penicillins or cephalosporins. This antibiotic therapy is essentially to relieve symptoms and can therefore cease when this has been achieved – usually in 5 to 7 days. Long-term chemotherapy for 2 to 12 weeks is occasionally needed for relapsing infections. However in these situations with chronic or relapsing infections surgical treatment is usually required for underlying obstructive disease. This is particularly true if secondary bladder stones, a rare though still well recognised complication of chronic sepsis, have occurred. This secondary bladder stone formation will fit into a vicious cycle of infection, stasis, stone and recurrent infection. In addition to further urine cultures therefore all men with more than one episode of 'cystitis' should have a plain X-ray to outline the bladder and reveal any bladder stones (Figure 3.3).

An IVP is not normally required but where recurrent infec-

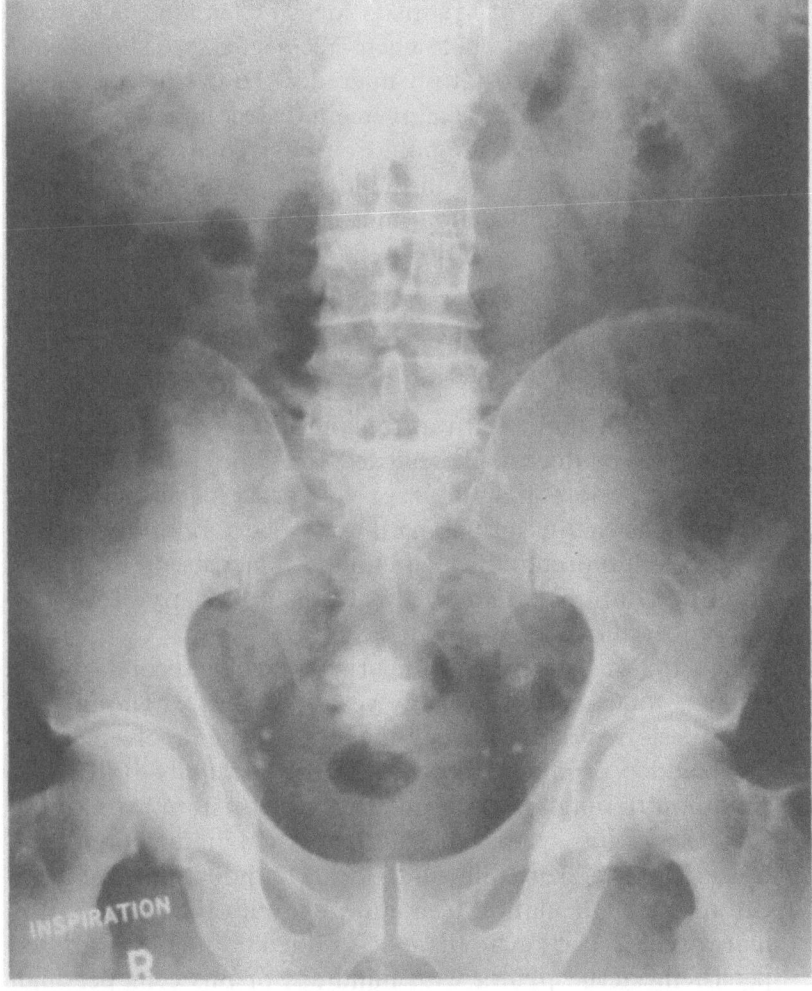

Figure 3.3   Bladder stone lying within thick-walled, dilated bladder

tion is present in association with obstructive symptoms an IVP will help to further define the degree of obstruction and the possibility of secondary effects such as stone formation or diverticula of the bladder.

A routine post-treatment MSU can be helpful but is not necessary where the patient's symptoms have resolved following appropriate treatment.

The management of cystitis is ideally placed in a general practice environment; but where recurrent sepsis presents, where subsequent prostatism underlies the cystitis or where the X-ray shows bladder enlargement or secondary stone formation, then the patient should be referred to a urologist[2]. Such a referral will result in the identification and release of bladder outflow obstruction and, if required, destruction of bladder stone.

Granulomatous cystitis

A final word about the rare but important granulomatous lesion of the bladder – tuberculosis[3]. Most major urology units will see no more than four or five cases of urinary tract tuberculosis each year making it a very rare condition indeed in any general practitioner's lifetime. An increase in the immigrant population should alert us to the possibility of urinary tract tuberculosis.

Tuberculous infection of the urinary tract is secondary to a primary focus occurring many years previously. Though the initial lesion is in the kidney the subsequent involvement of the bladder produces the cystitis which usually brings the condition to diagnosis. It is in effect another rare form of the 'chronic cystitis' syndrome. This time, though, infection is the cause. The bacilli are difficult to locate and the results of urine culture and inoculation techniques may not be reported for many weeks. The key to diagnosis is the finding of a so-called persistent sterile pyuria with hundreds of pus cells per high power field on microscopy. This urine finding combined with severe 'chronic cystitis' indicates urgent referral to a urologist for IVP and cystoscopy studies. These, in addition to the special urine cultures, will eventually enable the diagnosis to be made. Treatment is invariably hospital-based and involves elimination of the tuberculous disease and correction of the subsequent fibrous contractions of the urinary tract – particularly in bladder and ureter.

INFECTIONS OF THE GENITAL TRACT – PROSTATITIS

The involvement of the male genital tract with the urinary system is a most inappropriate anatomical association. The prostate by virtue of its position in the posterior urethra lies close to the bladder outlet where it can increasingly interfere with bladder emptying as hyperplasia develops secondary to ageing. Such obstruction, as mentioned above, producing as it does urinary stasis in the bladder, may result in intermittent and eventually marked 'cystitis'. But the prostate itself and the posterior urethra, through their genital associations with the ejaculatory ducts, may also result in infections loosely defined as 'prostatitis'[4]. This inflammatory and infective syndrome is to be clearly differentiated from the other prostate problem of primary obstructive disease – 'prostatism'.

The symptoms of prostatitis present in several ways (Figure 3.4).

(1) *Pain:* local perineal pain presents as a continuous debilitating ache, often extending to the lumbar, sacro-iliac and upper inner thigh areas.

(2) *Cystitis:* symptoms of frequency and dysuria will occur in association on occasion with haematuria.

(3) *Epididymitis:* this condition is thought to be due to reflux of infecting organisms either directly through or alongside the vas. This is in fact one of the commonest

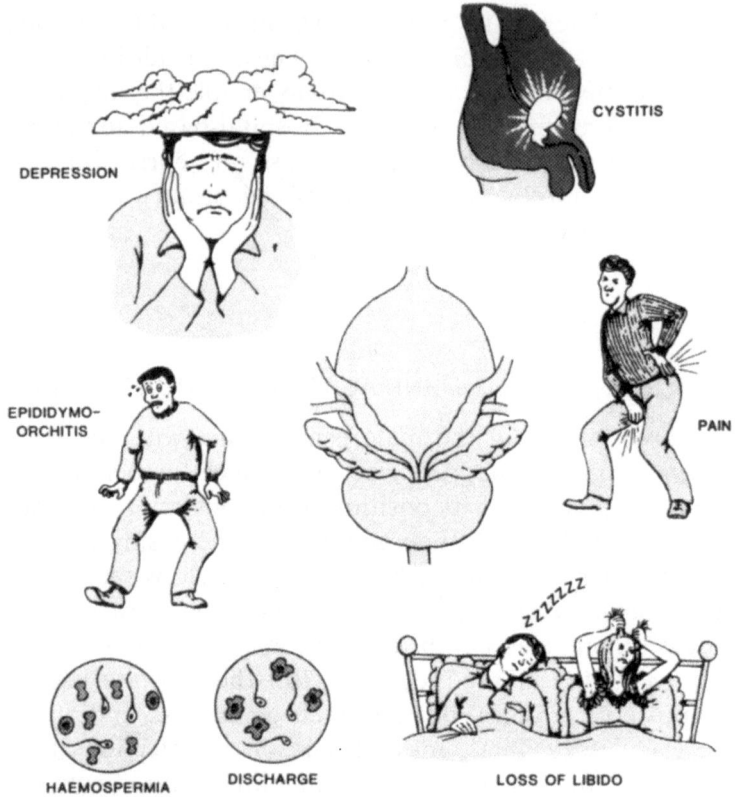

Figure 3.4   Presentation of prostatitis syndrome

presentations of epididymitis and prostatitis is indeed the only significant clinical cause of epididymitis.

(4) *Haemospermia:* fresh or old blood in the ejaculate can cause considerable alarm to the patient. However it is a totally benign condition and prostatitis is the only clinically significant cause of haemospermia.

(5) *Urethral discharge:* this is occasionally present and represents a move towards the more complex world of non-specific urethritis. This aspect of infection involves the

urethra proper and therefore lies more within the range of the genito-urinary physician.

(6) *Sexual:* decreased libido and painful ejaculation may present often causing sexual frustration for both partners.

(7) *Generalized:* there is often a vague malaise associated with prostatitis; the longer the symptoms have been present the more depressed or indeed more aggressive becomes the patient. In addition there can be anorexia, weight loss and sometimes even constitutional symptoms such as polyarthritis or conjunctivitis.

Prostatitis in all its many forms is an increasingly common diagnosis in young men. It traditionally affects tense, aesthenic men in their middle years (30 to 50 years) often in association with domestic or business stress, and in many cases related to sexual tension. Its cause is not clear. In a proportion of men organisms can be found in the prostatic secretion[5], which are, however, difficult to identify in many cases; their role as pathogens may be uncertain. The diagnosis is usually made on clinical grounds with a history as outlined above together with a finding of a tender, sometimes oedematous (so-called 'boggy') prostate on rectal examination. In many men the condition is associated with attacks every few months. In others the symptoms may be persistent usually with a continuous aching perineal discomfort as the main complaint. This in its extreme form is known as chronic prostatitis or prostatodynia. Such pain is morally and physically debilitating; some, fortunately few, patients become hopelessly depressed or even suicidal with such pain.

Prostatitis, though related to urethritis (i.e. non-specific urethritis), is not sexually communicable. Indeed most men with prostatitis have an almost complete cessation of sexual activity due to the combination of ejaculatory pain and loss of libido.

Investigation

Investigations are few. Urine cultures will exclude an underlying or masquerading urinary infection, particularly in patients presenting with cystitis symptoms. Prostatic secretions
can be obtained by prostatic massage producing the so-called
EPS (expressed prostatic secretion). This enables direct culture
of the prostatic fluid but still carries the risk of obtaining
urethral contaminants which are of no clinical significance.
The process of obtaining such prostatic secretion is itself
complex and unpleasant for the patient – it is therefore rarely
required in routine clinical practice. If it is examined, the
prostatic fluid may show changes in relation to pH and white
cell count that can be both diagnostic and prognostic for
the condition in difficult cases. Nevertheless, in the main the
diagnosis of prostatitis is made on clinical grounds. Patients
with prostatitis require long-term follow-up because of the
relapsing nature of the condition. Only after 12 months
freedom of symptoms can prostatitis be truly considered cured.
Monthly visits, especially for those on long-term chemotherapy, will help to maintain the patient's morale and confirm
his continued treatment.

No radiological tests are of value and the only reason for
referral to a urologist is in cases where diagnosis is difficult or
for those men who fail to respond to antibiotic therapy; more
aggressive surgical treatment may then be required.

Management

The condition has no significant mortality or morbidity. For
instance, no patient with prostatitis will necessarily be more
likely to have prostatism in later life. Do not, however, under-
rate the severe mental debilitation that prostatitis, especially
prostatodynia, can cause in some patients. These men benefit
from the dual management of hospital and general practitioners to see them through this difficult condition. Conservative treatment is based on empirical antibiotic therapy

using short-term (5 to 10 days) or long-term (6 to 12 weeks) courses of antibiotics. Virtually all antibiotics have been tried at some time but trimethoprim and tetracycline are most commonly used. With acute manifestations such as 'cystitis', urethritis or epididymitis a short course of therapy – 10 to 14 days – is all that is required. For haemospermia no treatment other than reassurance is necessary. For the chronic prostatitis patient with a painful prostate long-term therapy over a minimum of 3 months may be needed. Failure of antibiotic therapy following this should encourage the use of vigorous prostatic massage under general anaesthesia. This treatment is again somewhat empirical but it will help some patients. It can be performed as a day case but general anaesthetic is necessary as the treatment is both unpleasant and uncomfortable for the patient. It is presumed to have its effect through the emptying of the prostatic ducts of their retained secretions. It may be needed at intervals, however, and more recently attempts to ease prostatic pain more directly have involved the transurethral injection of the prostate with hydrocortisone and local anaesthetic. The early results of this treatment are encouraging. Other attempts to relieve the pain and urinary symptoms of prostatitis have included the use of ganglion-blockers to relax the posterior urethra. Spasm in this area is thought to contribute to most of the discomfort in these men. Results with this therapy have not been so impressive, mainly because of the often unacceptable side-effects of the ganglion-blockers.

Prostatitis remains a difficult condition to manage. However in general practice it is possible to control most of these patients' symptoms firstly by providing a full explanation of the condition coupled with a reassurance of its benign and ultimately self-limiting nature. This, as in young women with urethral syndrome, to which it has an uncanny relationship, is often the single most important treatment. Where symptoms persist aggressive antibiotic therapy will usually bring the situation under control. Only if this fails need the patient be referred to a urologist.

PRACTICAL POINTS

● Pyelonephritis is rare in the male and men with pyelone-phritis are ill. They do not usually present with lower tract symptoms but do have a high temperature and marked renal tenderness. Urolithiasis is a common underlying cause and hospital admission is usually needed.

● A normal MSU does not exclude a diagnosis of pyelone-phritis. The diagnosis therefore can be based on the history and examination alone.

● Management includes bed rest, oral fluids, and tri-methoprim or ampicillin for 14 days. If there is no improve-ment on home management within 48 hours hospital admission is indicated.

● A post-treatment MSU and an IVP should be arranged 2 to 4 weeks after the initial presentation in order to dem-onstrate a cure and to identify upper urinary tract obstruc-tion.

● Bladder infection in men is less common than in women but just as disabling. It is commonly a consequence of bladder neck obstruction due to prostatic disease.

● When bladder infection develops, symptoms can be sudden and include frequency, dysuria and haematuria. They are produced by detrusor (bladder muscle) irritability. When chronic the cause may be non-infective (e.g. malignant). 'Cystitis' symptoms should be differentiated from additional obstructive symptoms due to underlying prostatism. These include hesitancy, poor stream and terminal dribbling.

● Examination of men with cystitis is usually unrewarding as they are well but rectal examination is needed to identify the occasional malignant prostate. Urine culture is manda-tory and contamination is unusual.

● Trimethoprin and amoxycillin are the antibiotics of choice and are usually given for 5–7 days.

● A post-treatment MSU in men with cystitis is helpful but not necessary. In men with recurrent infection however a post-treatment MSU and plain X-ray are indicated. A post-treatment IVP is normally required only if renal infection has been suspected. It may also help to further define the extent of lower tract obstruction.

● Consultant help should be sought in the presence of recurrent sepsis prostatism (obstructive symptoms) and when X-ray shows bladder enlargement or secondary stone formation.

● Prostate infection (prostatitis) may need to be distinguished from prostatism (due to obstruction). There may be perineal pain, 'cystitis' symptoms of dysuria and frequency and haematuria and associated epididymitis.

● Prostatitis is an increasingly common diagnosis in young men and may be stress related. The diagnosis is usually made on clinical grounds. Urine cultures will exclude an underlying urinary infection. Radiological investigation is usually unhelpful. There are no significant long-term sequelae.

● Treatment is difficult and based on short or long-term courses of antibiotics commonly trimethoprim and tetracyline. Referral may be needed if aggressive antibiotic therapy is unsuccessful.

References

1. Kunin, C. K. (1979). *Detection, Prevention and Management of Urinary Tract Infection*. 3rd Edition, p. 4. (Philadelphia: Lea and Febiger)
2. Kunin, C. K. (1979). *Ibid.,* pp. 46–47
3. Narayana, M. S. (1982). Overview of renal tuberculosis. *Urology,* **19,** 231–237.

4. Meares, E. M. (1980). Prostatitis syndromes: New perspectives about old woes. *J. Urol.*, **123,** 141–147

5. Orland, S. M., Hanno, P. M. and Wein, A. J. (1983). Prostatitis, prostatosis and prostatodynia. *Urology,* **25,** 439–459

4

URINARY TRACT INFECTION IN CHILDHOOD

R. J. POSTLETHWAITE

Urinary tract infection is so common in childhood that it is easy to assume that it is of no significance. Fortunately the majority of children, even those with recurrent urinary tract infections, will have no long-term consequences, and as, in addition, any long-term consequences may be many years, if not decades, after the initial infection, the temptation to ignore urinary tract infections in children is strong. Despite the relative frequency of urinary tract infection (UTI) any single general practitioner's experience of it will be very limited, and this is particularly true of serious long-term sequelae. This further induces a false sense of security and, taking into account the difficulty of obtaining appropriate urine cultures, it would not be surprising if attitudes to the diagnosis and management of urinary tract infection are on occasion low key; perhaps best described as 'too little, too late'.

Yet it is certain that for a small number of children there will be very serious long-term consequences of urinary tract infections, and this is one of the largest potentially preventable childhood (and adult) problems. Present approaches to diagnosis and investigation are inconvenient but there is evidence that other countries are making a much more significant impact on this problem. In Sweden reflux nephropathy (chronic pyelonephritis) has virtually disappeared as a cause of renal failure in children. This is attributed to the high level of surveillance for UTI in children in Sweden[1].

The other danger with urinary tract infection in children is that there is great scope for over-diagnosis. This could result from relying on a clinical diagnosis, for example in assuming that all dysuria is due to urinary tract infection, using non-specific tests such as proteinuria as an indication of urinary infection, or accepting the growth found in a poorly collected, or poorly stored and transported specimen of urine, as diagnostic. In one recent report in only 9 of 33 urinary tract infections diagnosed on clinical grounds did the pre-treatment urine culture confirm the diagnosis[2].

INCIDENCE OF URINARY TRACT INFECTION

Urinary tract infection may be classified in a variety of ways. One major distinction which has been made is between symptomatic and asymptomatic bacteriuria. This distinction has little practical significance since long-term management is generally more closely related to the structural and functional characteristics of the patient's urinary tract rather than to the clinical presentation. From an epidemiological point of view, however, this distinction is important as any discussion must include patients with both symptomatic and asymptomatic bacteriuria.

Symptomatic bacteriuria

The apparent incidence of urinary tract infection will depend on the indications for urine culture, the accuracy of diagnostic techniques, utilization of health care facilities by the population, the number of patients at risk and the true incidence of UTI. Despite these problems a number of studies allow a fairly confident assessment of the incidence of symptomatic UTI in children. In Goteburg, Sweden, the community is relatively stable and all health care is obtained from a limited number of sites[3, 4], so that comprehensive information about symptomatic UTI in infants and children can be collected.

During the neonatal period the incidence of symptomatic urinary tract infection was 0.14 per cent. This excludes infants with myelomeningocoele, malformation of the external genitalia or obstructive lesions[3]. During the neonatal period there is a striking male predominance in the occurrence of all infections, including those of the urinary tract (see Table 4.1). The

Table 4.1 Sex ratio of symptomatic urinary tract infection

Age	Female:male
0–1 months	1 : 2.5
1–6 months	1.5 : 1.0
6–12 months	4.0 : 1.0
1–3 years	10.0 : 1.0
3–11 years	9.0 : 1.0
11–16 years	2.0 : 1.0

Source: references 3 and 4.

reason male infants have a two-fold greater incidence of sepsis, meningitis and urinary tract infections than female infants is not known. It is generally accepted that urinary tract infection in the neonate results from blood borne infection, and the increased incidence of UTI in the male appears to reflect the male infant's increased susceptibility to infection.

After the neonatal period the usual route of infection is ascending. Female predominance (Table 4.1) is usually attributed to the short female urethra but this is probably an oversimplification. The risk of symptomatic urinary tract infection in this series was 1:1000 boys per year and 2.8:1000 girls per year. The risk of symptomatic urinary tract infection

Table 4.2 Incidence of UTI in childhood

No. of infections	Incidence per 1000 children per year		Source
	Female	Male	
596	3.0	1.1	Winberg[4]
	(2.8)	(0.7)	(excluding neonates)
14	3.1	1.7	Dickson[5]
38	7.7	3.8	Brooks[6]
16	10.8	2.3	Loudon[7]

before the age of 10 years was 1 per cent in boys and 2.8 per cent in girls[4].

Data from some other studies of symptomatic urinary tract infection in children are summarized in Table 4.2. Dickson obtained three urine samples to make the diagnosis, the third sample being a suprapubic sample in infants[5]. Brooks and Houston[6] accepted a single urine as diagnostic and bag samples were collected from infants. This might explain the higher incidence of infections in their series. Collection technique is not clear in Loudon's paper but a single urine was obtained[7]. Thus the generally accepted incidence figures of 5 per cent for

Table 4.3 Recurrence of urinary tract infections

Age	Per cent recurrence	Time of recurrence
Neonates (both sexes)	26	Almost always within 1 year
Boys (< 1 year)	18	Almost always within 1 year
Girls (excluding neonates)	40	Two-thirds within 1 year One quarter within 1–4 years One tenth within > 4 years

girls and 1 to 2 per cent for boys for symptomatic urinary tract infection before the age of 10 years seem broadly correct and applicable to primary care.

Recurrences of infection are common (Table 4.3). In neonates of both sexes and boys under 1 year, recurrence of infection later than one year after the initial infection is rare. In girls (excluding neonates) late recurrences of infections are much commoner, though two-thirds occur within one year of the initial infection, a further 25 per cent of recurrences occur between 1 and 4 years after the primary infection, with 8 per cent of recurrences occurring more than 4 years after the primary infection.

The age distribution of symptomatic infections varies (Figure 4.1). In general hospital-based series have a higher incidence in the first year of life, 44 per cent in the Swedish report[4] compared with 11 per cent in one primary care paper[6]. Peak incidence in the primary care paper is 2 to 5 years. A

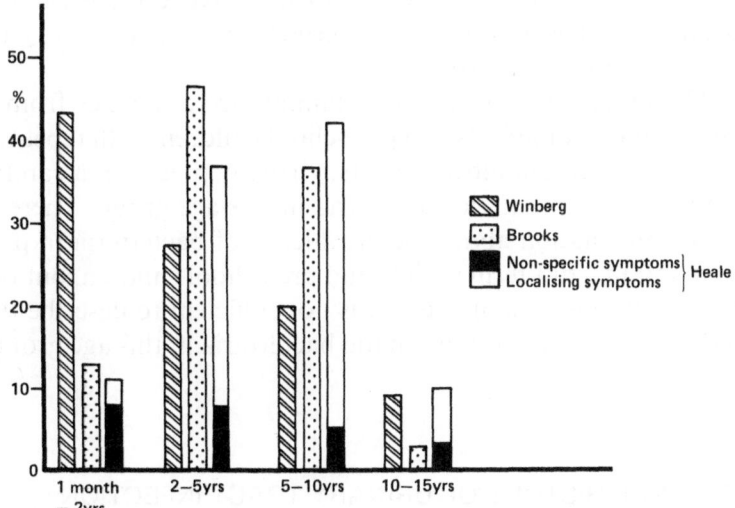

Figure 4.1 Age incidence of urinary tract infection from three sources: Winberg[4], Brooks[6] and Heale[8]. In the latter report the percentage of children presenting with specific and non-specific symptoms is indicated

series obtained from a casualty department in Australia has a similar age distribution to the primary care series[8]. The two most likely explanations of this difference are:

(1) selection in the hospital-based series – this is unlikely in the series quoted;
(2) under-diagnosis of urinary tract infection in the primary care series because of the non-specific symptomatology in the younger child.

Without age-specific incidence rates for all these reports it is not possible to say which of these, or other, explanations of these apparent differences is likely to be correct.

Asymptomatic bacteriuria

A number of studies of healthy school-aged children, using mid-stream voided samples of urine, have established the prevalence of asymptomatic bacteriuria at 1–2 per cent in girls and 0.3 per cent in boys[9].

The practical problems in obtaining urine samples from a large number of infants and pre-school children, with repeated sampling over a number of years, virtually precludes a careful study of asymptomatic bacteriuria in this age group. There is some information about the prevalence of bacteriuria in pre-term infants, full-term infants and pre-school children, but the information is incomplete and is not sufficient to describe the natural history of asymptomatic bacteriuria in this age group.

NATURAL HISTORY OF URINARY TRACT INFECTION

The development of renal scarring

It has long been recognized that there is a relationship between urinary tract infection and the entity 'chronic pyelonephritis'.

This label implies that it is 'chronic infection' that leads to renal damage and this impression, combined with the ease with which, in general, symptomatic infections are eradicated, suggested that patients with asymptomatic bacteriuria were the ones most at risk of long-term deterioriation. In studies of asymptomatic bacteriuria, no new scars developed after the age of 5 years in previously unscarred kidneys, even in the presence of persistent infection and/or ureteric reflux. Six per cent had progression of existing scars or new scar formation, but this progression was only seen in previously abnormal kidneys with severe reflux and persisting infection[9]. It is quite clear from these studies that asymptomatic bacteriuria on its *own* is not particularly important. Furthermore most damage has occurred by the age of 5 years and both reflux and infection seem necessary prerequisites for renal scarring. Though these studies suggest that asymptomatic bacteriuria is not the main mechanism for renal scarring and can be ignored in most children, in the young child with reflux or the older child with scarred kidneys and reflux there is potential for renal damage, and these categories of patients should be managed in the same way as patients with symptomatic urinary tract infection.

The relationship between scarring and vesico-ureteric reflux (VUR) is so well established that 'chronic pyelonephritis' is more accurately described as 'reflux nephropathy'. Forty per cent of adults with pyelonephritic scarring and over 90 per cent of children with pyelonephritic scars have reflux[10]. The incidence of reflux in normal children is not well established but is probably of the order of 1 to 2 per cent. It is unusual for children already under observation to develop new scars, but when new scars are observed they virtually only occur following further infections in the presence of continuing, usually severe, reflux[11].

Rolleston has demonstrated the importance of intra-renal reflux[12]. With intra-renal reflux, at cystography the dye passes not only into the pelvis of the kidney but into the renal substance (Figure 4.2). Follow-up studies showed that renal scars developed in the areas previously affected by intra-

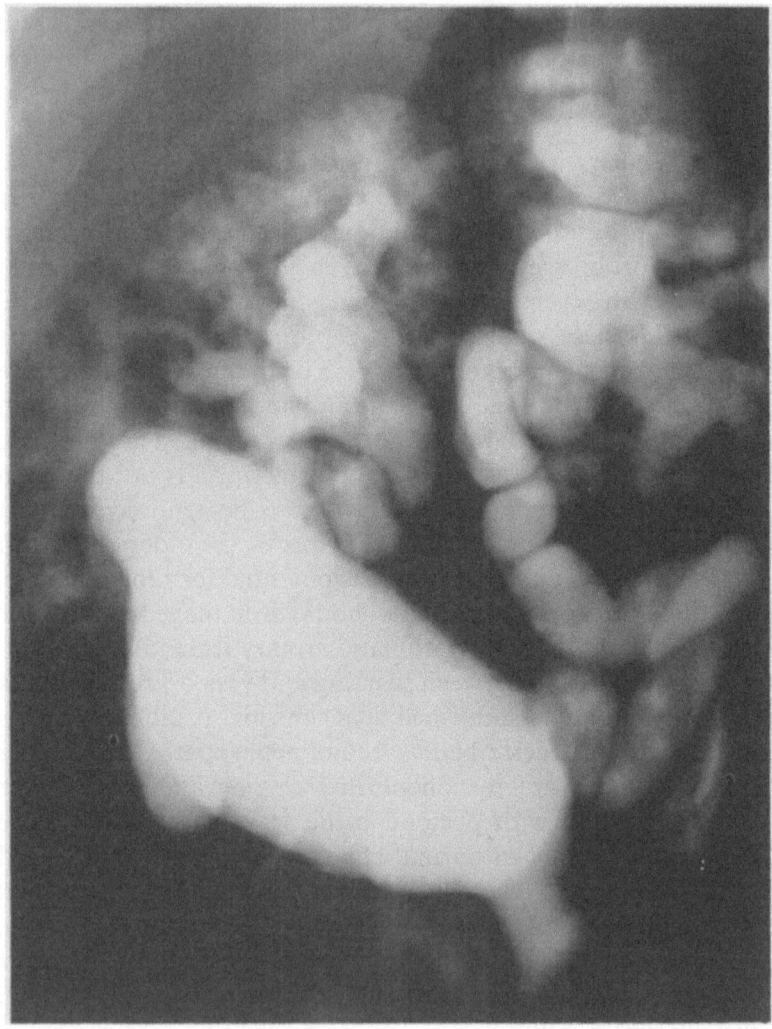

Figure 4.2   With intra-renal reflux the dye not only refluxes into the ureters and pelvis of the kidney but into the renal tissue itself. In this example virtually the whole of the renal tissue on both sides is outlined demonstrating extensive and bilateral intra-renal reflux

renal reflux (Figure 4.3). Ransley subsequently demonstrated that the morphology of the renal papillae determines whether or not intra-renal reflux will occur: he described so-called 'refluxing' and 'non-refluxing' papillae[13]. On the basis of these findings he suggested that in the presence of intra-renal reflux and infection near maximal damage occurs with the first urine

PRE   INFECTION   POST

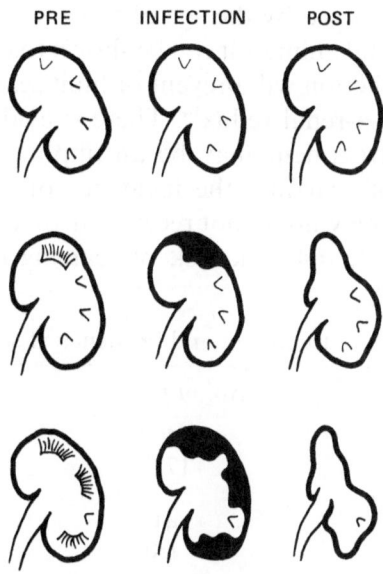

Figure 4.3 Schematic representation of the pathogenetic mechanism in the formation of pyelonephritic scars. Each row is read from left to right. In the top row though reflux is present there is no intra-renal reflux, so renal involvement with infection does not occur. In the middle row intra-renal reflux occurs into the upper pole of the kidney, so that with infection the upper pole is involved giving rise subsequently to scarring. In the bottom row virtually the whole of the kidney is affected by intra-renal reflux, so that with infection extensive damage occurs which is subsequently shown by almost complete scarring of the kidney. Both kidneys in Figure 4.2 would be expected to be damaged in this way if infection occurred. (From Ransley, P. G. (1982). Vesico-ureteric reflux. In Williams, D. I. and Johnston, J. H. (eds.), *Paediatric Urology*, 2nd Edn., pp. 151–166. (London: Butterworth Scientific) with kind permission)

infection. Reflux (except in the presence of a neurogenic bladder or obstruction) is generally agreed to be congenital. It predisposes to infection and hence most children with reflux will have an infection within the first two years of life. In the presence of intra-renal reflux this would lead to scarring. This would be one explanation of the finding that it is early infection that leads to renal damage, and would explain why most scarring has occurred by the age of 5 years.

In experimental animals it can be shown that early treatment of a urinary infection will prevent or limit scarring even in the presence of intra-renal reflux[14]. There is evidence in children that delay in treatment may be an important factor in the development of scarring; the incidence of scarring is much higher in children who do not receive adequate care at the first infection[15] (Table 4.4); the risk of scarring is twice as great

Table 4.4　Delay in treatment and incidence of scarring

	No. of patients	Per cent scarred
Adequate care*	440[15]	4.5
at first infection	178[16]	23
Inadequate care	41[15]	17
at first infection	68[16]	51

Adapted from references 15 and 16.
* Early diagnosis, investigation and treatment; follow-up after treatment.

in children with VUR who have recurrent infections before investigation compared with those investigated after a single infection[16] (Table 4.4). Only 1 of 116 infants had a scar on the initial intravenous pyelogram (IVP), whereas 25 per cent who were more than 1 year of age at the so-called 'first infection' had evidence of scarring, probably because of unrecognized and untreated early infection[15] (Figure 4.4).

Age, infection, reflux and intra-renal reflux are important factors in renal scarring. It may be that additional factors

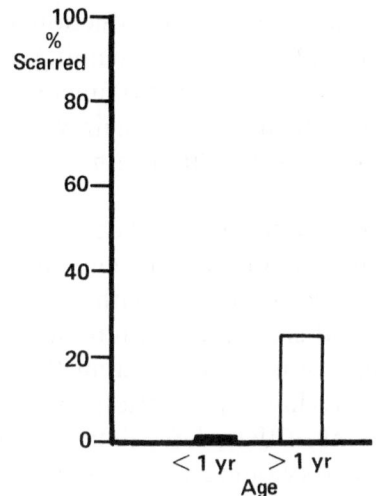

Figure 4.4   Age at first IVP and incidence of scarring[15]

might be necessary to account for renal damage, to potentiate damage, or (more unlikely) to provide other mechanisms for renal damage. Bacterial adhesion and P-fimbriated *E. coli* might be two such factors[15].

Later consequences

If renal damage is near maximal by the age of 5 years, why does end-stage renal failure not develop for many years? There are numerous possible mechanisms. Renal growth might be impaired so that renal function cannot increase to meet the needs of growth and subsequently of pregnancy. Renal damage due to infection might initiate secondary immunological processes which cause subsequent decline in renal function. Hypertension may develop many years after the initial renal insult and if severe, undetected or sub-optimally treated, could give rise to a secondary decline in renal function. There has been renewed interest lately in the concept that if renal mass is reduced without an appropriate reduction in dietary protein intake the hypertrophy in the remaining renal tissue can eventually give rise to declining renal function. These are some of the mechanisms which might explain why renal functional decline might be delayed for 20 or more years after the initial infection.

Another objection to the idea that early infection in children is the cause of later renal failure, is the apparent gap between the common problem of children with urinary tract infection and the rarity of end-stage renal failure due to reflux nephropathy. This difference is more apparent than real. Assuming that 5 per cent of girls have an infection some time in childhood and that 10 per cent of these have renal scarring, 5:1000 girls aged less than 10 years would have renal scarring. It is generally accepted that five to ten women per million population present yearly with end-stage renal failure due to reflux nephropathy[17]. This data is collected from dialysis returns and, therefore, largely affects women aged 15–55. Assuming a yearly incidence of 10 per million population, 300 women per million population will develop end-stage renal failure between the ages of 15 and 55 years, i.e. 0.3:1000 or about 1:15 women with pyelonephritic scarring. It is probable that further women will develop problems at an older age. Ignoring this possibility, the incidence between 15 and 55 years of end-stage renal failure in girls with pyelonephritic scarring would be about 7 per cent compared with the incidence of renal failure in the general population of about 0.075 per cent over the same period, i.e. end-stage renal failure will be 100 times commoner in this group.

In addition 25 per cent of children with pyelonephritic scarring will develop hypertension in childhood[18]. The number who develop hypertension in adult life is not clear but it is certain that the risk of hypertension developing persists for at least 10 years after the scarring event. Thus, if in addition to end-stage renal failure, hypertension and its consequences, and problems in pregnancy[19] are included in the assessment of the long-term consequences of pyelonephritic scarring, a very significant number of patients with scarring established in childhood will develop long-term problems.

SYMPTOMS OF URINARY TRACT INFECTIONS

The spectrum of symptoms in childhood urinary tract infection is very wide. Table 4.5 and Figure 4.5 summarize the infor-

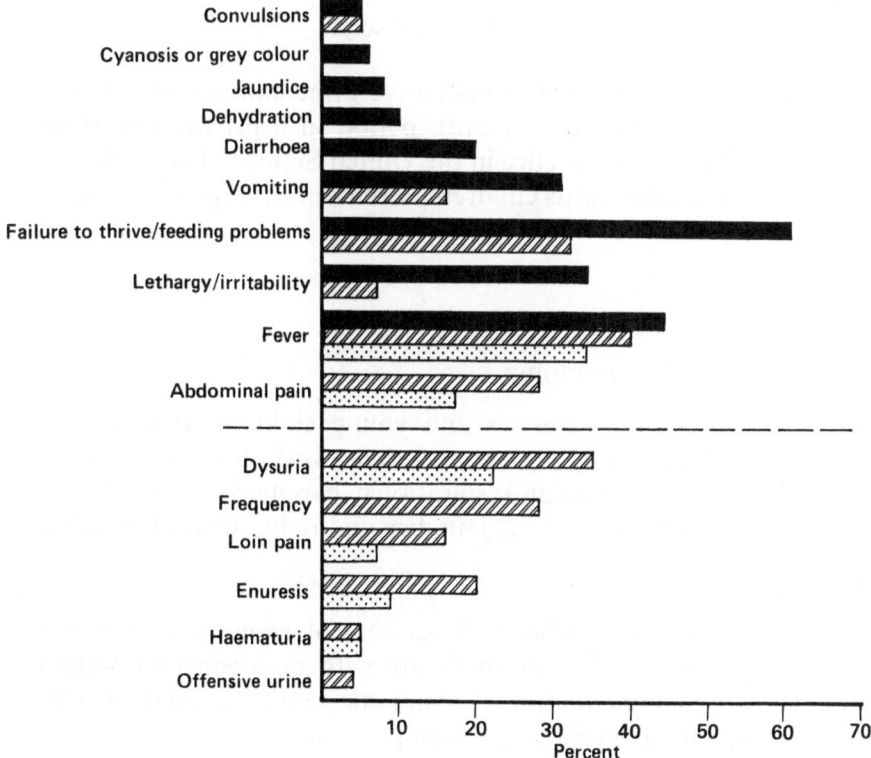

Figure 4.5   Symptoms of childhood urinary tract infection.
Sources: solid bars – Review article of neonatal urinary tract infections[20]
hatched bars – General paediatric department and accident and emergency department[8]
stippled bars – Private suburban paediatric practice[21]

mation about the symptomatology in childhood urinary tract infection from three sources.

(1) A review article on Neonatal Urinary Tract Infections[20]. This reflects the non-specific symptomatology in young children.

(2) A series collected over a 17-week period in a general paediatric department and accident and emergency department in Australia[8]. This is presumably much less selected than most hospital series.

(3) A series of 1000 consecutive urine cultures (112 infections) over a 30-month period in a private suburban paediatric practice in the United States[21]. This is clearly biased towards children presenting with specific urinary symptoms.

Non-specific symptoms

Clinical sepsis: Neonates and young children with urinary tract infection may present *in extremis* with shock, irritability, convulsions, irregular respirations, hypotension and hypothermia. Cyanosis, ileus, jaundice and reduced renal function may be present.

Failure to thrive: About 50 per cent of neonates and young infants present less dramatically with unsatisfactory weight gain or 'failure to thrive'. Anorexia, lethargy, feeding difficulties and irritability are often present.

Gastrointestinal symptoms: Vomiting and/or diarrhoea may occur at any age with urinary tract infection but is predominantly a symptom in the younger child. It may be so acute and/or severe as to produce dehydration or, if more long-standing, may lead to failure to thrive.

Fever is an important symptom of urinary tract infection at all ages. Any child of any age with a fever in whom there is not a clear cut diagnosis must have a urine culture taken.

Abdominal Pain: Children with acute or recurrent abdominal pain in whom the history and examination fails to reveal the source of the abdominal pain should have a urine culture taken: it is positive in about 6 per cent of children.

Specific symptoms

The classical urinary symptoms should immediately suggest the possibility of a urinary tract infection. The danger with these symptoms is to assume that they are diagnostic of urinary tract infection. Table 4.5 shows the percentage of children with various specific urinary symptoms (and some non-specific symptoms) who have positive urine cultures.

Table 4.5   Percentage of patients with specific urinary symptoms who have positive urine cultures

Loin pain	30
Haematuria	25
Recent wetting/daytime wetting	25
Frequency	21
Dysuria	12
Offensive urine	9
Vaginal discharge/irritation	7
Abdominal pain	6
Night wetting	3

Urgency, frequency, dysuria: A combination of these symptoms with or without suprapubic pain is commonly referred to as 'cystitis' and often assumed to be synonymous with bacterial urinary tract infection. The frequency/dysuria syndrome has multiple aetiologies, some obvious, some obscure. These are summarized in Table 4.6. External dysuria (pain felt as the

Table 4.6   Causes of frequency/dysuria in pre-adolescent girls

---

Local irritants
Bubble bath
Shampoo
Detergents (particularly biological detergents)
Fabric softeners
Tight-fitting garments, irritating fabrics, dyes in fabrics
Vulvo-vaginitis
Pinworm infestation

Systemic factors
Food, drink, medication (Vitamin C in some individuals)
Hypercalciuria (usually associated with haematuria)
Emotional stress (?)

---

urine passes over the inflamed labia) suggests vaginal irritation, while internal dysuria (pain felt inside the body) suggests a urinary tract infection. Considering the multiplicity of possible causes of frequency/dysuria in children it is not surprising that a number of reports have shown that only 20–30 per cent of children with these symptoms have bacterial urinary tract infection. Dickson[5], for example, found that only 6 of 34 children (18 per cent) with dysuria and frequency had urinary tract infections and he excluded children with obvious balanitis or vulvitis!

A combination of these symptoms is more suggestive of UTI. Thus 8.7 per cent of 92 patients with one of frequency, dysuria and loin pain had a proved infection, whereas 31.5 per cent of 57 patients with two or more of these symptoms had a proven infection[8].

Vaginal discharge/irritation: This merges into the frequency/ dysuria syndrome. There are often clues in the history (see above) and examination that suggest that the problem is vulvo-vaginitis rather than a UTI. It is surprising but useful to know that even in the presence of the vaginal discharge a single urine will exclude a UTI in 93 per cent of cases.

Haematuria: About 25 per cent of children with UTI have haematuria. In the majority of these, however, it is usually microscopic. In only about 5 per cent of children with urinary tract infection is the presenting symptom macroscopic hae-maturia; UTI is so much commoner than any other cause of haematuria in children, however, that at least 25 per cent of children with macroscopic haematuria will have a urinary tract infection as the cause. Again, bacterial confirmation is absolutely essential and will avoid much anxiety and unnecessary investigation.

Offensive smelling or 'strong urine' is a common complaint usually in infants or toddlers. Parents usually mean that the urine either looks dark, which indicates a concentrated urine, or the urine has an ammoniacal smell: this usually results from urea-splitting organisms from the bowel liberating ammonia from the urine and will happen if the nappy is left on the child, as might occur with poor hygiene or in a normal child overnight. It is usually easy to distinguish this ammoniacal smell, which rarely if ever indicates infection, from more abnormal smells, e.g. a fishy smell, which is associated with a *Proteus* urinary tract infection.

Enuresis: About 3 per cent of children who have never been dry at night-time have positive urine cultures, whereas the figure is 25 per cent for patients with a recurrence of enuresis or daytime wetting.

Loin pain: This has already been mentioned and again it is clear that bacterial confirmation is important. In a child with pyrexia, loin tenderness and a positive urine culture it is likely there is renal involvement in the UTI. The converse is not true: the majority of children with renal scarring from UTI have never had any illness remotely resembling this. Thus a facile division of urinary tract infections into 'benign' lower urinary infections and 'acute pyelonephritis' on clinical grounds is mistaken. The long-term outlook depends on the presence or absence of abnormalities detected in imaging rather than on

Table 4.7   Prevalence of infection in children with localizing and non-localizing infections

	No. of patients	Proven infection	Prevalence rate (%)
Non-specific symptoms	215[22]	17	8
	411[8]	18	4.4
Localizing symptoms	589[22]	108	18
	378[8]	54	14.3

Adapted from references 8 and 22. Figure 4.1 includes data on age distribution from reference 8.

any clinical assessment of the severity of the illness or the level of infection.

In summary, non-specific symptoms predominate in younger children; even within this age group the younger the child the more likely the child is to present acutely sick. In the younger age group widespread urine cultures will be required in children with non-specific symptoms. Even in the older child clinical diagnosis is still not possible though specific urinary symptoms are more common. In two series from Australia, one hospital based[8] and one primary care[22], only 14 per cent and 18 per cent of children with specific urinary symptoms had proven urinary tract infection (Table 4.7). The figures were even lower for children with non-specific symptoms – 4 per cent of the children in the hospital series and 8 per cent of the primary care series having a proven urinary tract infection.

DIAGNOSIS

Diagnostic signs

Pyuria: Undue importance is attached to the presence or absence of pyuria in the diagnosis of urinary tract infection.

Leucocyte excretion rates vary so that it is difficult to define normal levels. In addition pyuria may arise for many reasons apart from UTI (see Table 4.8).

Table 4.8   Some causes of leucocytes in urine

Inflammation of neighbouring structures, e.g. appendicitis
Urinary calculi
Healing of urinary tract after trauma or surgery
Glomerulonephritis
Chemical injury, e.g. analgesics
Severe dehydration
Leucocytes arising outside the urinary tract, e.g. vagina

If a low upper limit of normal is taken (10 cu.mm in uncentrifuged urine) there are few false negatives (0.6 per cent), but a large number of false positives (13.3 per cent)[5]. The results are even less clear-cut in children with recurrences or asymptomatic infections.

Proteinuria: It is all too common to have children referred with urinary tract infections on the basis of a positive dipstick test for protein (Albustix) in a febrile child. Treating albuminuria as a urinary tract infection verges on malpractice. Some of the numerous causes of both false positive and positive dipstick tests for urine protein are given in Table 4.9. A particular cause of confusion is the common occurrence of proteinuria in association with non-specific pyrexial illnesses. As, in addition, not all children with urinary tract infection have proteinuria this test is useless in the diagnosis of UTI.

Other tests: Of the numerous other tests which have been used in the detection of bacteriuria the nitrite test is the most useful. In the presence of significant bacteriuria with most gram-negative organisms, dietary nitrate in the urine is reduced to

Table 4.9   Causes of false positive and positive dipstick tests for protein

(i) *False positive*:
Gross haematuria, pyuria, bacteriuria
Alkaline urine
Dipstick left in urine too long
Contaminants and drugs (including antiseptics such as chlorhexidine)
Highly concentrated urine

(ii) *Positive:*
Postural proteinuria
Fever
Stress such as exercise or cold
Contamination of urine by vaginal secretions
Anatomical renal lesions
Glomerular causes (nephrotic syndrome, glomerulonephritis)
Tubular disorders

nitrite. Nitrite can be detected by the Greiss nitrite reaction which is available as a dipstick. False positives are uncommon but false negatives are a problem. Not all urinary pathogens produce this reaction and sufficient bladder incubation time is necessary. Though limited for these reasons a positive nitrite is some help in monitoring sick children at home.

Urine cultures: From the above discussion of symptoms and non-specific tests in the diagnosis of UTI it is clear that the diagnosis can only be established with certainty if bacterial confirmation is obtained.

Diagnostic levels

It is generally agreed that more than one clean voided urine is needed to diagnose a urinary tract infection. Kunin *et al.*[23] have shown that a single clean catch urine is positive in 7 per cent of children, only 1 per cent of whom are documented to have urinary tract infection on repeat sampling. Aronson[24] obtained simultaneous suprapubic urines and clean voided urines in children of different ages. In children aged 3–12 years four out of twenty children had positive clean voided urines with sterile suprapubic urines. From these observations it has been suggested that the probability of a urine infection is 80 per cent with a single clean urine rising to 96 per cent if two urine samples have been obtained.

Some authors have questioned these findings. Unfortunately Dickson's careful study does not indicate how many urines were positive on the first screening[5]. It is interesting that the percentage of definite infections in children with specifically urinary symptoms, presumably predominantly older children, in the two Australian surveys was very similar (14.3 per cent versus 18 per cent)[8,22]. The hospital survey obtained a second urine whereas the primary care survey relied on a single dip-slide specimen of urine. The situation might be different in children with non-specific symptoms, presumably pre-dominantly the younger children: the prevalence of definite infection was 8 per cent in the primary care series and 4 per cent in the hospital series, in the latter a second suprapubic sample of urine was obtained to confirm the diagnosis[8,22]. Mond et al.[25], achieved a remarkably low incidence of false positive urine samples taken in primary care, 1.1 per cent (14 out of 1259 specimens). The incidence of true bacteria was 0.4 per cent (5 out of 1259 specimens). Thus a single urine sample excluded bacteriuria in 98.9 per cent of specimens. Despite these reservations on present evidence, reliance on a single sample would expose four times as many children to urinary investigations as would be required if a second urine sample was obtained.

Erroneous results with bag collected urines have been even higher. Thus in the previously cited study 27 out of 62 bag specimens (43 per cent) were positive in infants under 18 months when all 62 suprapubic urines were normal[24]. For this reason bag specimens have fallen into disrepute in hospital practice. Again this has been questioned. Dickson found only

6.6 per cent false positives in 45 bag specimens[5]. This data suggests that a bag specimen in primary care is a useful initial screening test in the symptomatic infant, but it would be unwise to rely on this as a diagnostic test.

Another approach to this problem is to relate the findings in different series to the diagnostic tests used. Thus the series of Williams[22] and of Brooks et al.[6], show that even using a single urine culture there is a very significant number of children identified with serious renal pathology. The more urines obtained from infants with non-specific symptoms (a practice which seems essential) the more false positives will occur exposing infants to unnecessary investigations and follow up.

To summarize:

(1) It is not possible to make an accurate diagnosis of urinary tract infection on clinical grounds even in children with specific urinary symptoms.

(2) A single urine culture identifies a group of children who have significant renal pathology.

(3) Obtaining two urine samples will avoid unnecessary investigation in at least 75 per cent of children identified by a single urine culture.

Home urine culture techniques

Urine is an excellent culture medium, and unless it is plated out immediately (within 30 minutes) steps have to be taken to prevent bacterial multiplication.

Dipslides

These are a major advance in the diagnosis of urinary tract infection, and they would seem to be ideal for home testing of urinary tract infection[26]. They consist of a glass slide in a plastic container. On one side of the slide is MacConkey's medium and on the other a clear agar. Both culture media are inoculated by either dipping the slide in the freshly voided urine or preferably by holding the slide in the urine stream as the urine is being passed. Excess urine is then allowed to drain off. Culture then takes place within the sealed container by retaining it at the appropriate temperature. The results are read by comparison with a reference chart provided by the manufacturers (for full details see Chapter 1). Accurate results can be obtained after 24 h incubation at room temperature, though the results are rather more easy to read if the incubation takes place at 37°C. Positive slides can be sent to the laboratory for further bacterial identification and sensitivity testing if required. After initial incubation in primary care all (or selected) negative slides could be sent to a laboratory for further incubation if required, but this seems unnecessary. Since the bacteria are dispersed immediately onto a solid media at voiding, the problem of contamination virtually disappears and little or no preparation of the genitalia is required.

Other home culture techniques[27]

Storage and transport of the clean voided urine at 0–4°C will maintain the bacterial count for at least 48 h and probably longer. The urine must be chilled as soon as it is passed and maintained at this temperature till it reaches the laboratory. This must be very difficult in practice.

Boric acid preservation of urine samples is another accepted technique[28]. Not only does this method prevent multiplication of microorganisms but it maintains the urine protein pH and white cells. The volume of urine will influence the results (28 ml is the optimal volume), and the urine will subsequently require conventional bacteriological handling. Results will not be available within 24 h.

The Testuria filter paper method consists of a filter paper which has been dipped in the urine and is then used to inoculate a mini-plate. This is then incubated for 10–24 h at 37°C. This has also proved successful in primary care but is perhaps not as convenient or as easy to quantitate as the dipslide method. Cup and pad culture techniques similar to the dipslide technique are also available.

Any of these techniques could be used for home (or practice) urine culture, and it is for individual practitioners in consultation with their local bacteriologist to decide which method best suits their local needs, but the dipslide method seems almost ideal. Decisions about antibiotic therapy have to be made with some urgency, and with dipslides the general practitioner will have an initial result available in the practice within 24 h of urine collection 7 days a week. It would be difficult to achieve this with boric acid preservation, which seems the next most popular method, as the sample will need transporting to the laboratory (only during working hours) and the result communicating to the practice. Boric acid would seem to have an advantage on economic grounds as it costs about 5 p compared with 50 p for a dipslide. When costs of technician time and materials to prepare conventional plates are taken into account the economics are less clear-cut, and the additional cost of transport of samples and communication of results needs to be taken into account.

Obtaining urine samples

(1) *Under 2 years old*: The most convenient way of collecting urines is using a Hollister urine collecting bag (Figure 4.6). Some of the bacteriological worries about this technique have been discussed above.

The perineum is carefully cleaned with soap, rinsed with sterile water and dried thoroughly. The bag is attached securely to the perineum. It is preferable if the patient is kept upright, which is best achieved by sitting an infant on the mother's knee and by encouraging a toddler to run around without a nappy on. Immediately the urine is voided the bag must be removed. The urine is then either transferred to a sterile con-

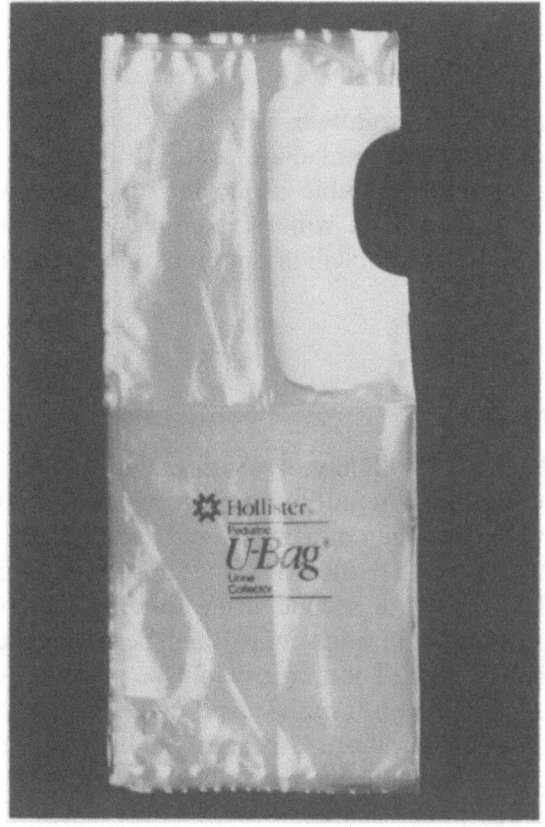

Figure 4.6   Hollister paediatric urine collection bag

tainer or poured over a dipslide. This is done by cutting a hole in a dependent corner of the bag (some bags have an aperture for this). The urine must not be decanted back through the entry hole.

(2) *Older children*: Wait till the child wants to micturate. The child then either stands over the toilet or in the bath with running water and the mother either collects urine in a sterile universal container or dips each side of the dipslide into the flowing stream of urine. Cleaning of the genitalia is probably not necessary but should be done for the second specimen.

Approach to diagnosis

Acutely sick children

These children will usually be neonates of infants with clinical sepsis. They require immediate accurate diagnosis and this will necessitate suprapubic aspiration of urine. Almost by definition these infants will need admission to hospital so there should be no problem in obtaining the appropriate urine sample.

Other infants

Most other infants will have less serious clinical illness and will not require immediate antibiotic therapy. An initial carefully collected bag specimen of urine should exclude a urinary tract infection within 24 h in the majority. Those with initial positive urines should have a second urine obtained by suprapubic aspiration and antibiotics could then be commenced whilst awaiting the result. Though it would be possible to perform these confirmatory suprapubic aspirations in general practice it would probably be more satisfactory to have an arrangement whereby these samples were obtained at the local paediatric unit on a day patient basis.

Assuming an incidence of urinary tract infection of 2.5/1000 patients under 2 years old per year (this figure is higher than most series), and that, for each with a definite urine infection, 10 children with symptoms have to have urines cultured, 25/1000 children under 2 years per year would have a urine cultured. The actual demand on the hospitals which would result from the strategy outlined above would be low, as would the numbers of 'unnecessary' suprapubic aspirations inflicted on the children.

Older children

This group presents no problem. Two clean voided urines should accurately diagnose an infection. In view of the good agreement between the results from conventional urine samples and from dipslides, two dipslides well collected should be at least as accurate as formal MSUs.

FURTHER INVESTIGATIONS

In 744 children investigated in a hospital series (Figure 4.7) 58 per cent had normal IVPs and micturating cystograms, 18 per

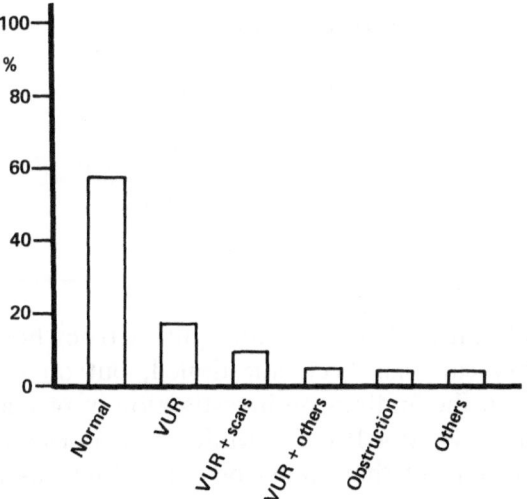

Figure 4.7 Findings on investigation of 744 children with urinary tract infections[16]

cent had vesico-ureteric reflux alone, 10 per cent had scarring plus reflux and a further 5 per cent had reflux plus other anomalies (obstruction, stones, duplex kidneys, horseshoe kidneys etc.). Thus 15 per cent had reflux with other anomalies. 9 per cent had other anomalies without reflux (scarring, obstruction, stones, etc.)[16]. These authors have shown that the incidence of scarring in children with ureteric reflux is higher the later the children are diagnosed, and this and similar data from Sweden has already been presented (Table 4.4 and Figure 4.4). Because of the high incidence of anomalies identified, and the evidence that late diagnosis is associated with a higher incidence of abnormalities, it has been accepted in hospital that all children should be investigated at the first infection.

Table 4.10 Incidence of anomalies in children with urinary tract infection

Number of Patients	Normal	VUR alone	VUR and other anomalies	Other anomalies	Source
744	58	18%	15%	9%	Smellie[16]
572	48	19%	33%		McKerrow[29]
38	–		8%		Brooks[6]
14	–		21%		Dickson[5]
125	64	36%			Williams[22]

The relevance of information gained from hospital series to primary care has been questioned, but on the available information the findings on investigation in primary care are very similar (Table 4.10). The McKerrow series is claimed not to be selected but there must be some doubt as the referral criteria were not formally ascertained[29]. 33 per cent had a renal anomaly with or without reflux and a further 19 per cent reflux alone. It is not clear in the Australian Primary Care series[22] whether all children had an IVP and a micturating cystogram (MCU), and neither can the children with reflux alone be separated out from those with reflux with other anomalies, but the results are remarkably similar to the other series. In Brooks' series[6] all the patients had IVPs, so that the figure of 8 per cent with anomalies with or without reflux is comparable to the 24 per cent in Smellie's data. In Dickson's study[5], too, not all patients had MCUs done but the study demonstrated a significant number of anomalies. The Australian paper[22] relates the prevalence of abnormalities to age at investigation, and shows that age does not influence the prevalence of anomalies for children under 10 years (Table 4.11).

Table 4.11   Incidence of anomalies related to age of investigations

Age (years)	Number of patients	Percentage with anomalies
0–5	50	34
5–10	54	31
10–15	12	8

Taken from reference 22.

Thus on currently available information the likelihood of finding anomalies in a primary care practice series is very similar to that in a hospital series, and age up to the age of 10 years should not influence a decision about investigation. Thus the same criteria can be applied to the investigation of children diagnosed in primary care as are used in hospital practice. Every child presenting with a UTI requires investigation to discover its aetiology, whether there is obstruction needing surgery, renal scarring or other abnormality of the kidneys, or reflux with its accompanying risk of future renal scarring.

Methods of investigation

IVP and MCU

The intravenous pyelogram (IVP) and micturating cystogram (MCU) offer the most informative and reliable primary investigations of the urinary tract, and a baseline from which to plan management and to which subsequent examinations can be related[30]. The IVP can demonstrate renal size, structure, function and calyceal pattern, the calibre of the ureters and bladder morphology. In addition spinal defects and an over-loaded large bowel can be seen. An MCU can demonstrate vesico-ureteric reflux (VUR) and sometimes intra-renal reflux, that is backflow of urine from the renal pelvis into the renal substance. These investigations do not need anaesthesia nor admission to hospital.

Newer imaging methods[30]

Ultrasound. This has the major advantage of being non-invasive and not involving radiation. It is useful in detecting hydronephrosis and other anatomical lesions, but is not yet a reliable method for detecting scars nor for serial measurements of renal size. As the presence of scars is the single most important feature determining long-term prognosis the ultrasound examination cannot be the primary investigation of urinary tract infection.

Radio-isotopes. The DTPA scan allows differential renal function studies to be made and is useful in assessing obstruction. The DMSA scan may prove to be the most sensitive means for the early identification of focal renal infection and thus of children needing intensive treatment, further investigation and follow up. The roles of radio-isotope imaging and ultrasound have not yet been clearly defined.

Programme of investigation

(1) Ultrasound as an initial investigation, particularly in infants in whom obstruction may be more likely to be important.

(2) An IVP in children of all ages with limited exposure.

(3) A cystogram in children
   (i) under the age of 5 years;
   (ii) over the age of 5 years but with recurrent infections;

(iii) evidence of renal scarring;
(iv) duplex or other abnormality on IVP;
(v)   family history of VUR or renal scarring.

VESICO-URETERIC REFLUX AND RENAL SCARRING

The main reason for treating urinary tract infections in child-hood apart from relieving symptoms is to protect the kidneys as far as possible from sustaining damage[30]. The incidence of scarring in children with UTI has already been discussed. Virtually all the children have ureteric reflux. Unfortunately scarring is usually already present when a child is first investigated. This may be either because the initial infection in early life was unrecognized and untreated, or because the initial infection was not investigated and followed up appropriately.

Recent studies[11] have shown that new scars can develop in previously normal kidneys or in normal areas of previously scarred kidneys. Fresh scarring can develop throughout child-hood. At least half of the new scars were in children over 5 years and in some children the scarring was extensive. Urinary tract infection was always present. There was significant and sometimes prolonged delay in diagnosis and treatment. VUR was usually present. The children often came from poor social circumstances aggravated by parental illness or separation[11].

VUR is usually present from birth and there is a strong familial association. It may be associated with other urinary anomalies such as duplex kidneys. Secondary reflux may develop in a child with an obstructed urinary tract.

Management

VUR without infection does not cause renal damage. Children with VUR treated with short courses of antibiotics show renal damage whereas in those given continuous low dosage prophylaxis the kidneys grow normally and no new scars develop[16]. In 85 per cent of undilated ureters and 40 per cent of dilated ureters reflux will disappear spontaneously. Thus a conservative regime can be recommended in the majority of infants and children. This consists of continuous low dose prophylaxis until reflux stops, with regular voiding and double micturition at bedtime and attention to bowels and fluid intake.

Surgical treatment

VUR can be corrected surgically and in the hands of an experienced surgeon this is a successful approach[30,31]. It is important for these operations to be carried out by surgeons experienced in paediatric urology. There are no clearly agreed indications for surgery. Surgery is more successful in moderate than severe reflux (as is medical management). 25 per cent of children continue to have infections after successful surgery and the risk of developing hypertension remains. Factors which influence the decision include:

(1) *Risk of breakthrough infections*: this is greater in younger children and in the presence of severe reflux. Each infection will carry a risk of further renal damage so that compliance is an important factor.

(2) *Chances of spontaneous resolution of reflux*: these are greater in the young child and in milder degrees of reflux.

(3) *Parental attitudes*: some parents are made very anxious by long-term prophylaxis, repeated investigations or the knowledge that a potential risk to the kidney remains. This anxiety can have profound effects on the child and is a strong indication for operation.

(4) *Risks of surgery*: the major risks are of failure to correct reflux as well as early or delayed obstruction at the vesico-ureteric junction. These risks are greater with severe reflux and possibly in early infancy. The tech-

nique used and the experience of the individual surgeon are also very important.

Thus indications for surgery in each individual case will vary; they depend on the patient, parents, physician and surgeon. Recurrent infection with renal involvement is the only clear-cut indication for surgery and, at the other extreme, operation should rarely, if ever, be considered in mild reflux. Fortunately controlled trials of surgery are currently under way which should clarify the situation[30].

TREATMENT OF ACUTE INFECTION

(The management of urinary tract infections is fully reviewed in reference 30.)

Choice of drug

If the child is ill treatment should not be withheld until a full bacteriological report is available (but appropriate urine cultures *must* be taken before antibiotic therapy). The choice of drug and route of administration will be influenced by a number of factors:

(1) The child's age and condition will determine whether or not parenteral therapy (and probably admission to hospital) is needed.

(2) The local patterns of bacterial sensitivities will affect antibiotic choice. The widespread use of a particular antibacterial drug either in primary care or in a hospital unit may result in an unusually high percentage of organisms being resistant to that drug.

(3) Any preceding history of antibacterial treatment, particularly with drugs which affect the bowel resistance

pattern, will influence therapy. If a urine infection arises in a child who has just received amoxycillin for a chest infection the likelihood is that amoxycillin will have eliminated all sensitive organisms from the bowel so that the urine infection is likely to be resistant to amoxycillin.

Taking these factors into account, an appropriate drug can be selected from Table 4.12.

Table 4.12   Drug treatments

Drug	Dosage ($mg\ kg^{-1}\ day^{-1}$)		Comments
	Therapeutic	Prophylactic	
Commonly used:			
Trimethoprim	4[a]	1–2[b]	Good for therapy and prophylaxis
Co-trimoxazole	24[a]	6–12	Good for therapy and prophylaxis
Ampicillin	50	—	
Amoxycillin	25[c]	—	
Nitrofurantoin	5	1–2[b]	Good for prophylaxis. Should not be used for therapy if systemically unwell or in uninvestigated urinary tract.
Nalidixic acid	50	15[b]	As for nitrofurantoin
Sulphonamide	100	20–25	
Less commonly used:			
Augmentin:			
amoxycillin	20[c]	—	
clavulinic acid	5–10[c]	—	
Cephadroxil	25		
Gentamicin	5–7.5(i.m)		

Total dose usually divided into 4 equal doses.
[a] Usually given twice a day; [b] usually given as a single dose at night-time; [c] usually given three times a day.

Dose and duration

It is usual to give full therapy for 7–10 days. A clinical response with sterile urine may be expected within 48 h. If there has been no response after 48 h the nature and sensitivity of the infecting organism should be checked and the appropriate drug prescribed. Single doses of antibiotics or 48 h of treatment have been used, mainly in adults, with satisfactory response. This approach is not advised in a child with a first infection with an uninvestigated renal tract. There is no evidence that courses of more than 14 days are more effective in eradicating infection or in reducing the recurrence rate, and they are more likely to result in the emergence of resistant bowel flora. Further antibiotic therapy depends on the findings on investigation.

FURTHER MANAGEMENT

Prophylactic antibiotics

The purpose of prophylaxis is to prevent reinfection of the susceptible urinary tract after the initial infection has been eradicated, and not to suppress inadequately treated infection. The ideal urinary prophylactic agent should be effective against urinary pathogens, it should be absorbed in the proximal part of the alimentary tract to minimize its effect on bowel flora as the emergence of resistant coliform organisms would render it ineffective, and it should have a high urinary excretion rate. It should be palatable, non-toxic and inexpensive. Administration in small tablet form or as a sugar free liquid preparation, is preferred, but if a liquid sweetened preparation is the only form accepted by the patient careful advice about dental hygiene should be given to the parents. Appropriate agents and dosages for prophylaxis are given in Table 4.12:

dosage is critical. Good therapeutic agents are not necessarily good prophylactic agents, and the prophylactic dose cannot be derived from the therapeutic dose.

Indications

Prophylaxis is appropriate in the following circumstances:

(1) following eradication of the presenting infection until appropriate investigations are completed in children under 5 years;

(2) in patients with VUR until the reflux resolves spontaneously or surgery is decided on;

(3) in the first year of life because of the vulnerability of the growing kidney, the lack of specific symptoms of UTI, and the problems of obtaining satisfactory diagnostic urine samples in infancy;

(4) in the older child, with normal IVP and MCU, prophylaxis may be indicated if there are frequent symptomatic UTIs, but it is likely when the prophylaxis is stopped that the infections will recur.

Breakthrough infections

This usually indicates poor compliance. The organism is usually resistant to the prophylactic agent, and the appropriate management is to change to therapeutic doses of another antibiotic, guided, ideally, by the antibiotic sensitivities. Following eradication of the infection low dose prophylaxis can be resumed, usually with a different agent as indicated by the urine (and hence faecal) culture. Frequent changes of prophylactic agent in a well controlled child are not indicated, and if dictated by breakthrough infections the cause of these relapses should be identified otherwise frequent changes of antibiotics will merely select out resistant organisms and give rise to infections which are difficult to treat.

Uncomplicated UTI

In the absence of any indication for prophylaxis (basically an older child with normal IVP and MCU) all that is required is treatment of each symptomatic infection. The overwhelming evidence is that the outlook for this group of children from a renal (if not symptomatic) point of view is excellent, and care should be taken to avoid producing any anxiety in the parents or child. Follow-up urine cultures should only be obtained when the UTI is symptomatic and the family should be positively reassured about the long-term outlook.

Follow-up urine cultures

Investigations at the outset will be orientated towards defining the risk of renal damage, and follow up urine cultures will depend on the findings on investigation. Regular urine cultures when asymptomatic are indicated in the patient with ureteric reflux (every 3 months) and in the first year of life (every 6 weeks irrespective of findings on investigation). All children should have urine cultures taken when symptomatic but therapy does not need to be delayed until the results are available. (This does not apply to the initial infection.) Some asymptomatic infections in children with normal investigations will be overlooked by this approach.

Other measures

Regular unhurried voiding at least every 2–3 h should be advised in all children, in addition double (or triple) micturition at night-time is important in children with reflux. This ensures that the bladder is emptied at least once a day. The child empties the bladder a second time (and sometimes a third) after an interval of 2–3 min until there is no residue of urine. Special attention needs to be paid to voiding at school as the child may not, for a variety of reasons, be happy or allowed to use the school toilet facilities.

An adequate fluid intake should be advised. Some children have no drink at breakfast, water is not always provided at school lunches, and the evening drink may have been cut out in bed wetters. Whilst ensuring an adequate fluid intake undue attention should not be paid to drinking habits.

Constipation is an important factor in urinary tract infection. Bowel habit should be enquired about and corrected if appropriate.

Follow-up

This needs to be co-ordinated between hospital and primary care. Adult specialists such as urologists have little concept of the special characteristics of urinary tract infection in children and approach the problem from an adult perspective. It would be helpful in paediatric departments if one paediatrician took a special interest in the problem. It is the author's impression that otherwise urinary tract infections do not receive the attention they should.

It is essential that continued follow-up, particularly urine cultures, are organized by the general practitioner. It is possible to organize follow-up urine cultures through the hospital but this is very much second best. The general practitioner is in a much better position to decide when to obtain urine cultures, he will be making decisions about antibiotic therapy which will affect prophylactic regimes, and he is in a position to advise and reassure the parents. The hospital's role is to advise about overall management, particularly re-investigation: this is particularly important in view of the development of newer imaging techniques.

Duration of follow-up

The indications for repeat urine cultures have already been discussed.

(1) Patients over 5 years with normal IVP and MCU should be followed for 2 years after the last infection.

(2) Patients under 5 years with normal IVP and MCU should be followed till age of 5 years or until 2 years after the last infection, whichever is the longer.

(3) Patients with reflux but normal kidneys should be followed until the reflux resolves and then can be dealt with as in (1) or (2).

(4) Patients with pyelonephritic scarring will require indefinite follow up:
  (i) Even with a single scar hypertension may develop in 10–25 per cent and the risk persists for at least 10 years.
  (ii) Contraceptive advice will be necessary. Oestrogen-containing pills may provoke hypertension, and unplanned pregnancies may be even less desirable than in normal young women.
  (iii) Particular care should be taken in pregnancy when there may be risk of hypertension and other complications.

Renal function should be checked in those with scarring and if abnormal repeated on a yearly basis (more often if renal function is severely impaired). Otherwise six monthly review for blood pressure measurement and Albustix testing of the urine is all that is required. Proteinuria may herald a decline in renal function and is an indication for full review.

SCREENING FOR URINARY TRACT INFECTION

Screening for urinary tract infection is not practical at the present time[30]. Screening programmes for asymptomatic bacteriuria have already been briefly discussed. Recognition that most damage has occurred by the age of 5 years has meant that screening of children on school entry has not been adopted while screening at earlier ages is beset by numerous problems. In addition the majority of children with pyelonephritic scarring will not have asymptomatic bacteriuria. Symptomatic bacteriuria is episodic and hence would not be detected by regular screening programmes. At present perhaps the greatest opportunity for prevention lies within the domain of primary care where early diagnosis might be facilitated by ready access to urine examination in any unwell child before antibacterial treatment is started.

WHAT TO TELL THE PARENTS AND CHILD

The natural history of urinary tract infection in children is now sufficiently well defined to allow parents to be given precise information about the risk to their child. One maxim which is frequently forgotten in a busy clinical practice is 'Don't talk in front of the children'. Even very small children will remember garbled scraps of information gathered from a conversation held between their parents and doctor. Often as time goes by the worst construction is erected on this information and major anxieties may not surface for many years.

The first concern of parents is that renal damage has or might occur. If the IVP and MCU are normal then parents should be specifically told that there is no risk to the kidneys. This message can often be re-inforced by showing the parents the X-ray films. This exercise also allows a brief description of normal urinary anatomy and is also useful when discussing children with abnormalities on imaging. The distinction between symptoms and long-term outlook needs to be emphasized. The child with normal investigations may have distressing recurrent symptoms which are difficult to control.

If reflux is present a brief discussion of how reflux predisposes to infection (by virtue of residual urine) and increases the risk to the kidneys (by carrying ascending infection up to the kidneys) is very useful, and allows the parents to understand the role of non-specific measures such as double micturition, and specific measures such as prophylactic antibiotics. The importance attached to the reflux will be varied according to the severity of the reflux, the presence or absence of renal damage, and the age of the child. A 5 year old with even moderate reflux who has a normal IVP, despite frequent infections, is unlikely to scar even if no action is taken, whereas the risks are much greater in a small baby.

A discussion of reflux naturally leads on to a discussion of the rationale of prophylactic antibiotics. Parents have been 'fortunately' indoctrinated to believe that antibiotics are bad for you, so that advice to use them on a long-term basis sounds like a dangerous heresy. The major worry is that in some way the antibiotics will 'lower the resistance to infection' and 'lead to infections that are more difficult to treat'. It is usually easy to allay these fears by careful explanation.

If there is any renal damage present the parents should be told the actual degree of renal impairment (if any) present. Actual figures for glomerular filtration rate related to normal, and to the level at which problems with renal failure are likely to occur, are easier to retain and discuss than vague statements such as 'a little kidney damage'. In the presence of any renal damage, the frequently unvoiced fear of parents is that the child's condition will suddenly (even overnight) deteriorate, and a careful discussion of the course of events in the unlikely circumstance that functional decline occurs is very reassuring for the parents.

Another unspoken fear is about dialysis: not only is there fear that this treatment may be necessary, but parents often feel that there is a lack of facilities and that as a consequence doctors avoid talking about the possibility. A specific discussion about dialysis is almost always necessary, even in parents whose child has normal investigations, and if after a few interviews it has not been raised spontaneously it is often wise to try to introduce the topic into the discussion.

The risk of hypertension will also need discussing. Again, figures such as 1:10 or 1:4 are more easy to appreciate than general statements. Parents need to know that hypertension may be delayed for years. The fact that at first it will be asymptomatic and easily treated needs stressing, as does the fact that if it is not detected because of failure of follow-up then further irreversible renal damage will probably occur before it becomes symptomatic.

For all children there will often be worries about everyday things such as teachers' attitudes to toileting, and other things such as dirty toilet seats as sources of infections. It is useful to encourage the parents to talk about these points so that sensible worries can be discussed and that taboos are not established.

The only involvement of children at first is to discuss their symptoms and prepare them for investigations which may be unpleasant. As they get older, certainly as they enter teenage years, they need to be involved wholly in the discussions because their anxieties will probably be greater than those of their parents. Erroneous decisions about careers might be made, anxiety might give rise to under-achievement at school, and they are rapidly approaching the age at which they will have to take responsibility for their own continuing care and will, therefore, have to understand in a balanced way the reasons for continuing observation.

PRACTICAL POINTS

● Although urinary infection in childhood is common the vast majority of children will have no long-term problems. This does not mean that infection is of no significance as for a small number there will be very serious and preventable long-term consequences occurring many years after initial presentation.

- Urinary infection in children is diagnosed too late so that irreversible renal damage is already established at presenentation.

- Urinary infection in children is overdiagnosed. Perhaps as few as one third of children who receive treatment have both clinical and bacteriological evidence of infection. Clinical evidence alone is unreliable when making a diagnosis. Dysuria has many causes. Non-specific tests such as proteinuria have no place in the diagnosis of urinary tract infection.

- Infection in the neonate is commoner in boys and results from blood-borne infection. After the neonatal period the usual route of infection is ascending and the customary preponderance of infection in girls is established.

- Both bacteriuria and vesico-ureteric reflux are needed to produce renal scarring and most damage has been done by the age of 5 years. Perhaps 1–2% of children have reflux. Delay in treatment may be significant in the development of scars. The significant aetiological factors are age, infection, vesico-ureteric reflux and intrarenal reflux.

- End stage renal failure may take years to develop; this could be because renal growth is impaired leading to functional embarrassment as a result of the demands of advancing years and of pregnancy. In addition secondary immunological processes may cause decline in renal function.

- About 10% of children with infection develop scars and one quarter of these develop hypertension in childhood.

- Symptoms of infection may be non-specific (sepsis, failure to thrive, gastro-intestinal symptoms, fever, abdominal pain) or specific (urgency, frequency, dysuria, offensive urine, haematuria, loin pain, enuresis). Only about one third of children with typical symptoms have urinary tract infection.

● The presence or absence of pyuria is relatively unhelpful in diagnosis. Proteinuria is of no value at all. Urine cultures are needed. Reliance on one MSU defines a population needing further investigation. Relying on two reduces that population by 75%.

● Hollister bags are commonly used when obtaining samples from children under 2 years. False positives are common. A better method (particularly in those over 2 years) is to obtain a clean catch specimen in a sterile container. Acutely sick children require suprapubic aspiration in hospital.

● All children under 10 years should be investigated after a first infection. Ultrasound is helpful in diagnosing hydronephrosis but not in defining scars. All children should have an IVP. A cystogram can be reserved for children under 5, children over 5 who have recurrent infection, evidence of renal scarring or other abnormality on IVP and a family history of VUR or renal scarring.

● Reflux disappears spontaneously in 85% of undilated ureters. Conservative regimes with low dose prophylaxis are usually recommended.

● Factors influencing the surgical treatment of VUR include the risk of breakthrough infection (greater in younger children and in the presence of severe reflux), the chances of spontaneous resolution (greater in the younger child and in milder degrees of reflux), parental attitudes (anxiety induced by chemotherapy and investigation) and the risks of surgery (failure is most likely when reflux is severe and in the younger patient).

● Treatment should not be withheld from an ill child while awaiting bacteriology. Appropriate drugs include trimethoprim, co-trimoxazole, ampicillin, amoxycillin, nitrofurantoin, nalidixic acid and sulphamonide. Therapy should be given for 7–10 days in the initial infection.

- Prophylactic therapy is usual in children under 5 until investigations are completed, in patients with VUR until it resolves or until surgery, in the older child if there are frequent symptomatic infections even when the IVP and MCU are normal, and in the first year of life.

- Follow-up is essential and the GP has a crucial role in deciding when to organize urine cultures. Patients over 5 years with a normal IVP and MCU should be followed up for 2 years after the last infection. Patients under 5 years with normal IVP and MCU should be followed until the age of 5 or until 2 years after the last infection, whichever is longer. Patients with reflux but normal kidneys should be followed until the reflux resolves and then are managed as above. Patients with pyelonephritic scarring require indefinite follow-up.

- Even with a single scar hypertension may develop in 10–25% and the risk persists for 10 years. Contraceptive advice is necessary. Oestrogen-containing pills may provoke hypertension. Pregnancy may require greater care. Renal function should be checked in those with scarring and if abnormal repeated at least on a yearly basis. Six-monthly reviews for blood pressure and proteinuria are usually required.

- Screening is not practicable at the present time.

References

1. Helin I. and Winberg J. (1980). Chronic renal failure in Swedish children. *Acta Pediatr. Scand.*, **69**, 607–611
2. Dighe A. M. and Grace J. F. (1984). General practice management of childhood urinary tract infection. *J. R. Coll. Gen. Pract.*, **34**, 324–327
3. Bergström T., Larson H., Lincoln K., and Winberg J. (1972). Studies of urinary tract infections in infancy and childhood. XII Eighty consecutive patients with neonatal infections. *J. Pediatr.*, **80**, 858–866
4. Winberg J., Andersen H. J., Bergström T. *et al.* (1974). Epidemiology of symptomatic urinary tract infection in childhood. *Acta Pediatr. Scand.* (Suppl 52), **63**, 1–20

5. Dickson J. A. (1979). Incidence and outcome of symptomatic urinary tract infection in children. *Br. Med. J.* **1,** 1330–1352

6. Brooks D. and Houston I. B. (1977). Symptomatic urinary infection in childhood: presentation during a four year study in general practice and significance and outcome at seven years. *J. R. Coll. Gen. Pract.,* **27,** 678–683

7. Loudon I. S. L. and Greenhalgh D. (1962). Urinary tract infections in General Practice. *Lancet,* **2,** 1246–1249

8. Heale W. F., Weldon A. F. and Hewstone A. S. (1973). Reflux nephropathy: presentation of urinary infection in childhood. *Med. J. Aust.,* **1,** 1138–1140

9. Verrier-Jones K., Verrier-Jones E. R. and Asscher A. W. (1986). Covert urinary tract infections in children. In Asscher A. W. and Brumfitt W. (eds.) *Microbial Diseases in Nephrology.* pp. 225–241, (Chichester: John Wiley and Sons)

10. Hodson C. J. and Edwards D. (1960). Chronic pyelonephritis and vesico-ureteric reflux. *Clin. Radiol.* **11,** 219

11. Smellie J. M., Ransley P. G., Normand I. C. S. *et al.* (1985). Development of new renal scars: a collaborative study. *Br. Med. J.,* **290,** 1957–1960

12. Rolleston G. L., Maling T. M. J. and Hodson C. J. (1974). Intra-renal reflux and the scarred kidney. *Arch. Dis. Child.* **49,** 531–539

13. Ransley P. G. and Risdon R. A. (1978). Reflux and renal scarring. *Br. J. Radiol.,* **14** Suppl., 1–35

14. Ransley P. G. and Risdon R. A. (1981). Reflux nephropathy: effects of anti-microbial therapy on the evolution of the early pyelonephritic scar. *Kidney Int.,* **20,** 733–742

15. Winberg J., Bollgren I., Kälennius *et al.* (1982). Clinical pyelonephritis and focal scarring: a selected review of pathogenesis, prevention and prognosis. *Pediatr. Clin. N. Am.,* **29,** 801–814

16. Smellie J. M. and Prescod N. (1986). Natural history of overt urinary infection in childhood. In Asscher A. W. and Brumfitt W. (eds.) *Microbial Diseases in Nephrology.* pp. 243–245. (Chichester: John Wiley and Sons)

17. Kincaid-Smith A. (1983). Reflux nephropathy. *Br. Med. J.,* **286,** 2062–2063

18. Smellie J. M. and Normand I. C. S. (1979). Reflux nephropathy in childhood. In Hodson J. and Kincaid-Smith P. (eds.) *Reflux Nephropathy.* pp. 14–20. (New York: Mason Publicity)

19. Becker G. J., Ihle B. U., Fairley K. F. *et al.* (1986). Effect of pregnancy on moderate renal failure in reflux nephropathy. *Br. Med. J.,* **292,** 796–798

20. Pascual J. F. (1974). Neonatal urinary tract infection. *Contrib. Nephrop.,* **15,** 41–46

21. Leape, L. L. and McEachen W. H. (1974). Office urine cultures in paediatric practice. *Postgrad. Med.,* **56,** 177–182

22. Williams C. M. (1976). Urinary tract infection in children: General Practice survey. *Aust. Fam. Physician* **5,** 340–344

23. Kunin C. M., Southall J. and Paquin A. J. (1960). Epidemiology of urinary tract infections. A pilot study of 3,057 school children. *N. Engl. J. Med.* **263,** 817

24. Aronson A. S., Gustafson B. and Svenningsen N. W. (1973). Combined suprapubic aspiration and clean-voided urine examination in infants and children. *Acta Paediatr. Scand.,* **62,** 396–400

25. Mond N. C., Grüneberg R. N. and Smellie J. M. (1970). Study of childhood urinary tract infection in General Practice. *Br. Med. J.,* **1,** 602–605

26. Arneil G. C., McAllister T. A. and Kay P. (1973). Measurement of bacteriuria by dipslide culture. *Lancet,* **1,** 94–95

27. Ogra P. L. and Faden H. S. (1985). Urinary tract infections: an update. *J. Pediatr.,* **106,** 1023–1029

28. Porter I. A. and Brodie J. (1969). Boric acid preservation of urine samples. *Br. Med. J.,* **2,** 353–355

29. McKerrow W., Davidson-Lamb N. and Jones P. F. (1984). Urinary tract infection in children. *Br. Med. J.,* **289,** 299–303

30. Smellie J. M. and Normand I. C. S. (1986). Management of urinary tract infection. In Postlethwaite, R. J. (ed.) *Clinical Paediatric Nephrology.* pp. 372–393. (Bristol: Wright)

31. Ehrlich R. M. (1982). Vesicoureteric reflux: a surgeon's perspective. *Pediatr. Clin. N. Am.,* **29,** 827–834

5

URINARY TRACT INFECTION AND THE ELDERLY

S. L. CHOUDHURY and J. C. BROCKLEHURST

Urinary tract infection is a very common finding in the elderly and in general practice between 1 and 6 per cent of consultations concern symptoms suggesting urinary tract infection (UTI); they occupy a significant portion of general practitioners' time. Various reports indicate infection in the urinary tract in elderly women to be around 20 per cent of those in the community rising to over 30 per cent amongst those in hospitals and old people's homes. It rises by about 1 per cent per decade until the 40s and at about twice that rate throughout the rest of life in women. In males bacteriuria is rare in childhood and throughout adult life until the seventh decade when it rises to around 15 per cent (in the community) and is found predominantly among men who have undergone urinary tract instrumentation. Despite this very high prevalence of significant bacteriuria in the elderly, the condition has received relatively little attention when compared with the young and with women of childbearing age.

CLINICAL PRESENTATION

The signs and symptoms of inflammation produced by urinary infection may extend from the renal cortex to the urethral meatus. Infection may be predominantly at one site or at more than one site. Upper urinary tract infection consists predominantly of pyelonephritis. Lower urinary tract infection may involve 'cystitis', prostatitis, urethritis or there may be significant bacteriuria without any evidence of tissue involvement (bladder bacteriuria).

The classical presenting symptoms of urinary tract infection are often the same in the old as in the young, including fevers, rigors, vomiting, pain in one or both loins radiating to the iliac fossa and suprapubic area (in upper tract infection) and associated with the signs of tenderness and guarding over the renal angle and lumbar region. In lower tract infection the signs are those of the 'dysuria-frequency syndrome' – urgency, frequency, dysuria, strangury (painful desire to pass urine though the bladder is empty), scalding and incontinence. The urine may have an unpleasant odour and appear cloudy. However in old age the clinical picture is often atypical, an extremely common presentation being with mental confusion and none of the classical symptoms (although tenderness and guarding may be discovered). Similarly, dysuric symptoms, incontinence (including stress incontinence) and nocturnal frequency commonly occur in the absence of urinary tract infection and indicate other aetiologies.

Very occasionally the first evidence of urinary infection in old age is metastatic infection such as osteomyelitis, septic arthritis, endocarditis, subdural empyema, septic pulmonary embolism and endophthalmitis. These indicate haematogenous dissemination which is occasionally spontaneous but more likely to be associated with manipulation of the urethra, prostate or bladder as part of a surgical procedure or with indwelling urinary catheters.

The greater part of bacteriuria in the elderly, however, is asymptomatic (i.e. covert infection). It may also present as

isolated fever (pyrexia of unknown origin) with apathy or
vague symptoms such as loss of appetite, fatigue, dizziness,
increasing immobility, falls and abdominal discomfort.

Thus, any of this huge spectrum of atypical symptomatology
which cannot be explained on any other basis requires examination of the urine for cells and organisms.

ASSOCIATED CONDITIONS

Faecal incontinence with poor perineal hygiene is sometimes
causally associated with urinary tract infection and this is
particularly the case among old people in institutions,
especially those suffering from senile dementia. No correlation
has been reported between bacteriuria and socio-economic
factors in the elderly.

Prostatic infection is sometimes the source of urinary tract
infection in elderly men. Prostatic infection itself is usually
heralded by characteristic symptoms of urinary irritation and
frequency with terminal dysuria. These may be superimposed
on the symptoms of long-standing prostatism and outflow
obstruction. Fever is unusual unless there is an established
prostatitis with focal inflammation and possibly abscess formation. Such infection may be complicated by epididymitis
and may then be expected to show a systemic reaction with
pyrexia. In men with suspected urinary tract infection, therefore, digital examination of the prostate per rectum is essential.
Tenderness will be marked in the presence of prostate infection
making exact examination of the gland difficult. In such cases
excretion urography could also be carried out to define the
condition of the kidneys and note any residual urine.

Acute pyelonephritis in the elderly may present non-specific-
ally or with the systemic disturbances noted above. Tenderness and guarding in the renal angles and lumbar region are
usual.

'Cystitis' and urethritis are often asymptomatic although

suprapubic tenderness may be present and the urine may be cloudy and foul smelling.

Infection can be associated with other abnormalities within the urinary tract. These include bladder outlet obstruction, renal or bladder calculus, presence of diverticula and analgesic nephropathy. Infection in this situation is often recurrent and may be associated with chronic pyelonephritis with impaired renal function. In these 'complicated' cases control of infection is therefore particularly important.

DIAGNOSIS OF URINARY TRACT INFECTION IN OLD AGE

The overwhelming majority of cases of urinary tract infection (particularly in the community) are due to gram-negative aerobic bacilli and the diagnosis is based on the colony count of more than 100 000 colonies per ml of urine. It must be emphasized, however, that even in cases of infection with gram-negative coliform organisms, no absolute count precisely confirms or excludes the diagnosis of a urinary tract infection

Table 5.1   Some factors influencing bacterial counts in old age

---

(i)   Method of collection and processing of the sample
(ii) State of hydration
(iii) Frequency of micturition
(iv) Presence of obstruction
(v)   Administration of antimicrobial agents

---

and quantitation of bacteria depends upon a number of factors (see Table 5.1). Moreover, a bacterial count of more than 100 000 organisms per cm^3, in a single random voided specimen is evidence of infection with an 80 per cent degree of confidence. Anaerobic bacteria may occasionally be present particularly in the setting of structural abnormalities in the urinary tract. Rarely, other microorganisms such as fungi, virus, tubercle bacillus and parasites may be the cause and no established criteria for diagnosis in these cases are yet available.

Since there is such a high prevalence of significant bacteriuria in old people, both in the community and in institutions, it is clearly impracticable to diagnose and treat all such patients. In fact, asymptomatic bacteriuria in old age is generally regarded as a benign condition not requiring treatment. However, the atypical methods of presentation are so very common in old age that a urinary culture is one of the most commonly required tests. The urine should also be examined for bacteriuria in patients with renal failure or with active glomerular damage as indicated by proteinuria.

COLLECTION OF URINE FROM THE ELDERLY

It is sometimes thought that obtaining a 'clean catch' specimen of urine from old people is difficult and often impossible and there is no doubt that this is the case in confused patients who are bedridden. Suprapubic aspiration of urine has been recommended but this is not an easy procedure in the elderly, particularly in those with whom it is most difficult to get a clean catch specimen. In such patients, therefore, (and particularly in women) it is often perfectly reasonable to use a catheter briefly inserted to obtain the necessary urinary specimen.

In those who can co-operate a suitable specimen of urine can be obtained in women by cleansing the vulva with a soap solution and tap water and drying it with a sterile swab. In males the foreskin should be fully retracted and the glans penis cleaned in a similar fashion. Antiseptic solution should not be used for these purposes. Collection of a mid-stream specimen of urine is a difficult procedure to follow, particularly for the elderly women. Collection of any 'clean catch' specimen is usually satisfactory for diagnosing UTI in the elderly. Under no circumstances should the urine that is to be studied bacteriologically be an aliquot taken from a larger container such as urine bottles or a bed pan, nor should the urine specimen be brought from home in a container. Contamination may indeed be less common in elderly women because of reduced vaginal secretion and the virtual disappearance of pubic hairs. Incontinent patients, of course, require catheterization to obtain an appropriate specimen.

If a prostatic source of infection is suspected in men then the 'three specimen' collection could be used. The first 5 to 10 ml of urine represents the urethral sample. Ideally micturition should be stopped just before it is complete and prostatic massage carried out, followed by collection of the final specimen which should then contain prostatic fluid. However, this procedure can be difficult (see Chapter 3).

The avoidance of delay in despatching the specimen to the laboratory is equally important in the old as with other age groups and if this is not possible then refrigeration of the specimen at 4 to 6°C for up to 48 h is acceptable. Use of a maintenance preservative like boric acid or of a dip inoculum culture may be helpful (see Chapter 1).

Several different culture methods are available for enumeration of bacteria. The direct counting procedure still seems to be the simplest and least expensive available method. A number of chemical tests have also been developed for detection of significant bacteriuria but are not entirely reliable (see Chapters 1 and 4).

ORGANISMS

E coli accounts for 80 to 90 per cent of community-acquired infections followed by *Klebsiella, Proteus, Enterobacter, Pseudomonas, Staphylococci* and *Streptococci.* In hospital, however, *E. coli* accounts for only about 50 per cent of cases and the other wide variety of less frequently occurring organisms accounts for the rest of nosocomial infections and these organisms tend to be resistant to commonly used antimicrobial agents (see Chapter 1). A mixed growth should not be dismissed in old people although it is helpful to repeat this culture if possible. However, infection due to more than one organism does occur in the presence of underlying structural abnormalities and certainly with an indwelling catheter.

Unusual organisms

Unusual organisms are more often found in diabetic patients and those receiving corticosteroids or immunosuppressive drugs. Infection with L-form bacteria has been found in some patients with recurrent infection after a presumed successful course of treatment. *Staphylococcus saprophyticus* is now recognized as the cause of about 20 per cent of infection in young women, but is rare in old age.

Direct examination of urine for acid-fast bacilli has little value in suspected cases of tuberculosis in the urinary tract since other non-pathogenic acid-fast bacilli may sometimes be found. Culture on appropriate media is therefore necessary to diagnose this disease. Tuberculosis may present simply with urinary frequency and nocturia.

While viruses may be found in the urine in the course of many systemic viral infections, it is difficult to distinguish between passive glomerular filtration of these organisms from the blood and true renal infection.

Candida organisms are occasionally isolated from elderly individuals but their presence rarely gives rise to concern although their clinical significance is uncertain. Isolation of *Histoplasma capsulatum, Coccidioides immitis, Blastomyces dermatitidis* and other primary pathogenic fungi, however, would suggest a true infection.

Renal lesions are common due to schistosoma and other parasitic infestation in endemic areas.

PREDISPOSING CAUSES OF URINARY TRACT INFECTION IN THE ELDERLY

Most urinary tract infections in women are caused by the ascent of organisms from the perineum. Haematogenous infection is rare. Faecal incontinence and poor perineal hygiene thus encourage infection. In old age, urinary stasis due to outflow tract obstruction provides a persistent and effective medium for bacterial multiplication. Prostatic hypertrophy (and carcinoma) account for the great majority of infections in elderly men. In women, vaginal prolapse even of slight degree increases the possibility of urinary tract infection. Other predisposing causes are stones in the urinary tract, neoplasia and necrosis of the renal papillae. The presence of residual urine may also be due to an imperfectly emptying neurogenic bladder. Vesico-ureteric reflux seems to be less common in old age than in children and its role in the pathogenesis of pyelonephritis is not known.

Papillary necrosis may occur in chronic pyelonephritis, diabetes mellitus, vascular disease and analgesic abuse and these conditions often present with the superimposed infection. The part played by instrumentation and prostatic infection have already been referred to. Infection may occasionally arise in localized infarcts of the prostate.

In old age, immunological vigour wanes and this may be a further factor predisposing to urinary tract infection. While it is generally understood that elderly diabetics have a higher prevalence of urinary infection there is some conflicting evidence on this score. Diabetic autonomic neuropathy, however, may lead to degrees of retention making infection more likely.

Association of urinary tract infection with prostatectomy may be due to the removal of a prostatic secretion which is thought to have some antibacterial effect. In women, the role of oestrogen deprivation leading to atrophic vaginitis as a predisposing factor for infection has not yet been fully explored.

LOCALIZING THE SITE OF URINARY TRACT INFECTION

In most old people there is no need to localize the site of infection in uncomplicated symptomatic and asymptomatic bacteriuria. A relatively small group of elderly patients with urinary tract infection and a high recurrence rate with distressing symptoms, or patients with suspected urinary infections with evidence of progressive renal function deterioration may be considered for investigations for localizing the site of their urinary infections. These patients are more difficult to cure and require longer treatment, so it is helpful to localize the infection in these cases if possible. Relapsing bacteriuria (the rapid recurrence of infection with the same species of organism as was present before therapy) is more frequently associated with upper urinary tract infection whereas reinfection (recurrence of urinary tract infection with a different organism) is more common in lower urinary tract infection. The former provides another group in whom it is useful to localize the site of infection. At least this will eliminate unnecessary prolonged courses of potentially more hazardous antibiotics in treating patients who do not have upper urinary tract infection.

Table 5.2   Invasive and non-invasive methods of localizing UTI

  (i) Invasive:
      Renal biopsy
      Ureteric catheterization
      Bladder washout
      Differential culture of prostatic secretion

 (ii) Non-invasive:
      Measurement of maximum urine osmolality
      Water loading test
      Measurement of urine fibrinogen/fibrin degradation product
      Serum antibody determination
      Pattern of response to treatment
      Imaging techniques

Unfortunately, no method of localizing urinary tract infection (see Table 5.2) is entirely satisfactory. There are excellent reviews of the tests available to identify the site of urinary tract infection[1,2]. Direct techniques are hazardous and cannot be justified in many elderly patients. They are lengthy, uncomfortable, expensive and may produce bacteraemia. Imaging studies and determination of antibody-coated bacteria (ACB) in the urine are probably the most useful methods currently available.

WHO SHOULD BE TREATED?

Most bacteriuria in the elderly is clinically silent. The question immediately arises as to whether one should look for bacteriuria in patients who are not complaining of any distress, particularly since there is a strong body of opinion that asymptomatic bacteriuria in old people should not be treated – it is a relatively benign condition and does not affect renal function nor diminish life expectancy. Such opinion does not recommend screening and treatment of asymptomatic bacteriuria in the elderly unless there is evidence of obstruction or back pressure. The toxic side effects of drugs, risk of super-infection, the cost and the high rate of recurrence, all argue against treatment. Moreover, the high prevalence of bacteriuria in the elderly, both in the community and in institutions, suggests that it is impracticable to treat and continue treating all such patients.

One population study showed that a high proportion of women with bacteriuria lose this spontaneously as time goes by. The rate of such turnover is about 20 to 25 per cent annually and a similar number acquire infection during the course of the year.

Conflicting reports, however, argue that it is unwise to view asymptomatic bacteriuria as harmless even in the absence of risk factors for renal disease. A higher rate of deteriorating renal function has been shown in the elderly who are bacteriuric compared with those who are not. A series of studies from Athens following a population over a number of years showed that those with bacteriuria died sooner even after correcting for age and weight. This was among ambulant residents in a large home for the elderly and applied to both sexes and all ages above 70.

These controversies must lead to anxieties, in some elderly patients with urinary tract infection, about the risk to their renal function and in such cases careful clinical assessment and reassurance is necessary. In general, the major determinant of urinary infection causing renal function deterioration is the presence of structural and neurological lesions in the renal and outflow tracts. If urograms or other imaging techniques indicate abnormalities then surgical referral is important. If, on the other hand, no abnormalities are demonstrated the physician can be reasonably optimistic about the long-term prognosis. Frank renal insufficiency is not the chief cause of death in bacteriuric elderly patients – if it were this would be recognized and recorded. It is possible that associated diseases such as dementia and other diseases of the central nervous system, or indeed any debilitating illness which reduces life expectancy may also predispose to the development of bacteriuria. For instance, patients with brain failure usually have a lower level of personal hygiene and more faecal soiling of the perineum.

As a general rule, a single short-term course of therapy should be given to all patients in whom bacteriuria is encountered for the first time. If symptoms are relieved by this therapy then further treatment may be necessary should reinfection or relapse occur. If there is no effect on symptoms, or if the patient is asymptomatic, no further course of treatment should be given even in the case of reinfection or relapse.

It has been suggested[3] that aggressive treatment with antibiotics should be used in all elderly patients in some situations (Table 5.3).

Table 5.3   Circumstances in which aggressive antibiotic treatment is proposed[3] for elderly patients with UTI

(i)   Following an initial episode of proved bladder infection
(ii) Infection in the presence of renal insufficiency (creatine clearance <40 ml min^{-1})
(iii) Infection in the presence of glomerular damage (moderate to heavy proteinuria)
(iv) Febrile patients with upper urinary tract infection (especially if lithiasis present)
(v)   Suspected gram-negative septicaemia with UTI
(vi) Acute; non-specific symptoms with UTI (confusion, fatigue, dizziness, falls)

MANAGEMENT OF UTI IN THE ELDERLY

Once a decision to treat the infection has been reached the following system of management may be useful.

General advice

Many patients limit their fluid intake because of the symptoms of frequency and they – and indeed all elderly subjects with urinary tract infection – should be advised to increase their fluid intake and to practise frequent micturition to keep their bladder as empty as possible. This should contribute to the dilution of bacteriuria and the frequent washout of the organisms.

Treatment of the acute attack

In symptomatic infection the severity of symptoms frequently demands treatment before bacteriological findings and the sensitivity pattern of urinary pathogens are known. In these circumstances ideally a urine specimen should be sent to the laboratory and an antimicrobial agent prescribed based on the likely causative organism. On the other hand, if there are few

or no symptoms it is best to wait for results of urinary culture
before initiating therapy.

In deciding which antimicrobial agent to use, various factors
should be borne in mind (Table 5.4). Whatever drug is used a
second specimen of urine should be sent for culture 4 to 6
weeks after completion of the initial course to ensure that the
infection has been truly eradicated.

Table 5.4   Factors influencing the choice of antimicrobial agent

 (i) Community or hospital-acquired infection?
 (ii) Potential side effects of drug *versus* severity of illness
(iii) Is the regime:
        simple
        free of toxic effects
        cheap rather than expensive
        appropriate to the level of renal function
(iv) Patient's previous experience of a particular drug

It is generally assumed that optimal results are obtained by
keeping as high a level as possible of the antibacterial agent
in the urine for 1 week. On the other hand, however, clearing
of bacteria has been described both with lower levels of antimicrobials and shorter periods of treatment. First line drugs
in the community are likely to be sulphonamide, trimethoprim,
or a combination of these. Broad-spectrum penicillins, nitrofurantoin and nalidixic acid are also useful for primary treatment. In hospital-acquired infections the cephalosporin
derivatives are very effective for elderly patients and well tolerated.

If the treatment is appropriate the symptoms will subside
within 48 h in the great majority of cases and the urine becomes
sterile within a few days. Generally, the treatment is given for
5 to 7 days. Patients with suspected acute pyelonephritis who
remain toxic, develop bacteraemia, or remain febrile for more
than 96 h after the onset of antibiotic treatment should be
suspected of obstructive uropathy or perinephric abscess and
require evaluation by imaging techniques and uro-surgical

advice. On the other hand, continuation of mild symptoms without fever or other systemic upset for 4 or 5 days after starting antibiotics is an indication for reculturing the urine and reviewing the antibacterial agent.

Parenteral antibiotics are required for patients with bacteraemia and those with pyelonephritis which is associated with systemic symptoms such as shaking, chills, sweats and fever with tachypnoea.

Since most organisms causing UTI are derived from the faecal flora, the widespread use of antibiotics – particularly in institutions – leads to a high incidence of resistant organisms in the bowel flora. This may be the reason for the high degree of recurrent urinary tract infection with multiple resistant bacterial strains in patients in geriatric hospitals and wards.

Although a week's course of treatment is generally prescribed, many patients never complete this since they stop taking the drug once symptoms have subsided. There may therefore be an advantage (particularly as far as side effects and cost are concerned) in considering a shorter course of therapy. Numbers of studies have shown that even a single dose of antibiotic may be effective in the treatment of uncomplicated symptomatic lower urinary infections (e.g. ampicillin (2 g), sulphamethizole (1 g), double strength co-trimoxazole). This may be particularly useful in patients with an uncomplicated 'dysuria-frequency syndrome' but in general a course of at least 3 days is recommended (see Chapter 2). In domiciliary practice a 3-day treatment regime with amoxycillin has been described as superior to 1-day treatment in 'dysuria-frequency syndrome' but no difference in result was found between a 3-day and a 10-day course of treatment. Co-trimoxazole repeated on two successive nights (total of six tablets) has also been described to be as effective as treatment with fourteen or more tablets. It remains uncertain as to whether single dose therapy will prove generally adequate in acute uncomplicated infections in the elderly.

In most cases of acute 'dysuria-frequency syndrome' antibiotics are rarely needed for more than a week. In chronic cases prolonged courses of antibiotics (more than 2 weeks) using the same or a series of agents has not been shown to have any advantage and are likely to raise the risk of toxicity and resistant organisms.

Prophylaxis

The place of long-term prophylactic treatment has to be considered in a relatively small number of elderly patients with recurrent infection which is symptomatic and for which several attempts at short-term antibiotic therapy have failed to prevent the recurrence. Resistant organisms are more likely to be encountered in such patients and treatment, therefore, should be given by bacteriological monitoring. A standby course of antimicrobial agents may be given to such patients so that they can start treatment at the onset of symptoms, immediately after preparing the dipslide inoculum. In such cases antibiotics (including ampicillin, sulphonamides, cephalexin, nitrofurantoin, co-trimoxazole, etc.) are usually started in full dose and slowly reduced to one or two tablets a day. Urine cultures should be taken every 3 months or so and the withdrawing of this regime after 6 months or longer must be attempted.

In the past, urinary antiseptics have been used on a long term prophylactic basis but the success rate is low and side effects common, particularly in the presence of impaired renal function.

Management of complicated infections

Complicated infections are likely to be those associated with anatomical malformations of the urinary tract, obstruction to urinary flow, analgesic nephropathy, ischaemic scarred kidney, chronic pyelonephritis, and calculi. Resistant organisms are much more likely to be found in these situations since multiple courses of antimicrobial agents will probably have been used.

Such organisms are often difficult to treat and are resistant to commonly used antimicrobials. Another problem is the urea-splitting properties of *Proteus* leading to a very alkaline urine which will diminish the effectiveness of most antibacterial agents (other than aminoglycosides and erythromycin). Other pathogens such as *Klebsiella,* micrococci and T strain of myco-plasmas may also produce urease and raise the urinary pH. The production of struvite calculi is more likely in these cir-cumstances. In the presence of such organisms it is not easy to acidify the urine with the commonly used oral acidifying agents.

Patients with complicated infections require short-term therapy for acute episodes and prophylactic antimicrobial treatment is contra-indicated.

Wherever possible surgical relief of any obstructing factor in the renal tract should be attempted in such cases. In the case of renal calculi, however, this is not always successful since minute particles of stone may remain in the urinary tract and favour persistent infection with urea-splitting organisms. The long-term effect of urethral dilation and ureteric reim-plantation for intractable 'cystitis' in women has been attempted but is generally disappointing.

The role of L-form bacteria in complicated urinary infection is uncertain but if it is suspected a course of erythromycin may be used as it acts on cellular synthesis rather than cell wall production.

Management of UTI in the presence of renal failure

In the presence of renal failure the problem is to maintain an effective concentration of drugs in the urine without so prolonging the half-life of the drug systemically that side effects follow. In severe infections antibiotics whose excretion is related to glomerular filtration rate (such as the amino-glycosides) are usually given in a loading dose and subsequent dose schedules are individually adjusted. Ideally this should be on the basis of serum concentration although the serum creatinine level may provide an approximate guide and of course symptoms of toxicity must be watched for closely. The drugs which are mainly excreted through non-renal routes are not particularly effective for urinary infections especially in the presence of renal failure.

Measurement of serum level of antibiotics is particularly recommended when drugs with a limited range of critical serum level are used. For example, gentamicin requires a concentration above $5 \mu g \, ml^{-1}$ and below $10 \mu g \, ml^{-1}$ to ensure a bacteriocidal level in the serum without systemic toxic effects. Diuretics may increase toxicity of aminoglycosides and also the cephalosporins. Tetracyclines (with the exception of doxy-cyline and minocycline) are particularly toxic at high serum levels and should always be avoided in the presence of renal failure.

In general drugs such as sulphonamides, nalidixic acid, ampicillin and most other penicillins which are excreted by the kidney, but whose toxic effects are not directly related to their serum concentration, can be used in the presence of renal failure with safety in their normal dose. Problems associated with these drugs are those of skin sensitivity. Co-trimoxazole and most of the cephalosporines (with the exception of cephaloridine due to its nephrotoxic effects) can be used either with less frequent doses or by decreasing doses after the loading doses.

Drugs such as erythromycin, lincomycin, doxycycline, sodium fusidate, clindamycin, etc., which are excreted largely by extra-renal routes may be used for tissue infections but do not give good urinary concentration and are therefore of little value in the treatment of UTI in the presence of renal failure.

Treatment of prostatic infection in the elderly

The prostate is an obvious source of urinary infection in the elderly and this is particularly so in the presence of prostatic calculi, when mixed infections are quite often seen.

Acute bacterial prostatitis responds to most antibacterial agents and co-trimoxazole is recommended for initial therapy. The management of chronic prostatitis however is more difficult (see Chapter 3). Commonly used antibacterial agents are lipid-insoluble, bound to protein, highly ionised in plasma and fail to penetrate prostatic fluid. If they do succeed then the high acidity of the fluid may render them ineffective. Drugs which are most useful in chronic prostatitis are co-trimoxazole, erythromycin, oleandomycin, tetracycline and clindamycin. Three months treatment may be required and even such prolonged courses may not eradicate infection in all patients particularly in the presence of calculi. The only solution then in attempting to control recurrent UTI is a complete prostatectomy.

Recurrent infection in men is also associated with infective triple phosphate or struvite calculi. Wherever possible such stones should be removed or dissolved by agents such as acetohydroxamic acid (an analogue of urea which acts as a competitive inhibitor of urease).

Complicated infections in elderly women

The factors associated with recurrent infection in women are shown in Table 5.5. In recurrent attacks of symptomatic bacteriuria, the first line of treatment may be to provide several courses of drug to be taken immediately when symptoms recur. But a kit should also be provided for dip inoculum culture and sensitivity tests of the organisms, which the patient should use immediately before taking the drug. There is no convincing evidence that extending the duration of therapy or increasing the intensity of the drug will reduce the incidence of reinfection in women particularly when it is confined to the bladder.

The use of prophylactic treatment in these circumstances is best avoided wherever possible since it will not affect the biological defects which predispose to the recurrent infection

Table 5.5   Factors associated with recurrent UTI in elderly women

---

  (i) Infrequent voiding
 (ii) Uninhibited neurogenic bladder
(iii) Persistent colonization of the introitus and vaginal vestibule
(iv) Relatively high pH of vaginal secretion in menopausal women
 (v) Enhanced adherence of organisms to introital mucosal cells
(vi) Absence of cervico-vaginal antibody
(vii) Thinning and atrophic changes of the vaginal and peri-urethral
     epithelia

---

and side effects can be a problem. Such prophylactic therapy should be tried only in women who experience multiple disabling flare-ups. In addition the use of very potent new antibiotics on a prolonged basis may cause profound changes in the intestinal flora with the development of resistant organisms in the bowel and the development of superimposed infection of the urinary tract from these organisms. If prophylaxis is to be attempted then low doses of drugs such as nitrofurantoin (50 mg nightly), co-trimoxazole (in decreasing doses – even to one tablet weekly), trimethoprim, methenamine mandelate and hexamine hippurate (Hiprex) or hexamine mandelate (Mandelamine) given at night when the bladder emptying is less frequent. Long-term treatment with nitrofurantoin can, however, lead to the development of pulmonary infiltrates, chronic pulmonary fibrosis and polyneuritis. In some patients long-continued sulphonamide has been reported to produce Stevens Johnson syndrome.

Intra-vaginal oestrogen has been used with some success in post-menopausal women with recurring UTI. *E. coli* rarely occur in the vaginal introitus at a pH of less than 4.5 (the normal vaginal pH is around 4). 'Cystitis', if present, is first treated with an appropriate antibacterial agent and the patient put on suppressive therapy appropriate to the organism colonizing the vagina. This is continued while oestrogen is given in a unit dose delivering 0.3 mg of oestrogen. This is given intra-vaginally for 7 days and then every second day for 7 days, and finally every third day until vaginal culture reverts to normal (i.e. that seen in premenopausal women). The dose is then titrated to the lowest necessary to maintain a vaginal pH of 4.0–4.6. This is usually one dose every 4 to 7 days.

Surgical procedures such as urethral dilation and internal urethrotomy have also been claimed to be successful in the treatment of recurrent UTI but there is no clear evidence of this in elderly women so far.

Elderly patients with UTI who should be referred to a hospital

Four groups of patients who should be referred for specialist treatment are shown in Table 5.6.

Table 5.6 Elderly patients who should be referred for a specialist opinion

---

  (i) Ill patients who do not respond to conventional simple measures and treatment with antimicrobial agents after five to seven days
 (ii) Ill toxic patients with fever, rigor, hypotension, vomiting and who are unable to tolerate oral therapy and patients with suspected septicaemia or peritonitis
(iii) Patients with complicated UTI
(iv) Symptomatic patients with infection from unusual organisms resistant to commonly used antibiotics

---

PROBABLE LONG-TERM EFFECTS OF UTI IN THE ELDERLY

Renal function

The effect of asymptomatic bacteriuria in the elderly on renal function remains controversial. The majority of patients who die from renal failure suffer from glomerulo-nephritis rather than chronic pyelonephritis. Some authors suggest that asymptomatic bacteriuria is only harmful if it is associated with raised blood pressure, obstructive uropathy and other complications. Retrospective studies in women have shown no difference in urine concentrating power, serum creatinine or blood urea compared with age-matched controls who did not have a past history of UTI. Similarly, follow-up of adult bacteriuric women over a period of 5 years did not reveal a rise of serum urea or creatinine levels greater than that which might have been accounted for by ageing.

On the other hand, there is some evidence that asymptomatic bacteriuria and pyelonephritis may be associated with deteriorating renal function. A correlation between an autopsy demonstration of pyelonephritis and a post mortem bacterial count of urine obtained by bladder puncture has been described. Several studies have also shown a relationship between asymptomatic bacteriuria and significant impairment in tubular capacity, glomerular function and renal circulation.

This question therefore appears to remain unresolved.

Bacteriuria and hypertension

The relationship between bacteriuria and hypertension is also not certain. Some studies have shown a positive relationship between elevated blood pressure and bacteriuria. A positive relationship between bacteriuria and hypertension in hospitalized patients has been described but the same work did not show it in old people living at home. This suggests the possibility of other factors inducing both of these conditions and since both are very common it is difficult to know whether or not there is a causal relationship and, furthermore, eradication of infection has not so far been shown to lower blood pressure. Bacteriuria is particularly common in immobile aged patients with cerebrovascular disease and encephalopathy and these also are more likely to have hypertension as a primary problem.

Bacteriuria and mortality

The uncertainty concerning the relationship between asymptomatic UTI and both renal failure and hypertension also extends to its effect on mortality. One general population study on women aged 15 to 84 years indicated that the duration of infection was related to its ultimate effect on mortality. Where a correlation has been shown between asymptomatic UTI and mortality, the cause of this relationship has not generally been demonstrated. Deaths from gram-negative septicaemia usually occur in hospitals and frank uraemia due to urinary infection has rarely been identified as the chief cause of death. Many terminal diseases such as cerebrovascular disease and brain failure both diminish life expectancy and also predispose to bacteriuria. It is suggested that in elderly patients non-recovery during the course of debilitating illness may be due in part to the reduction in the kidneys' capacity to maintain plasma tonicity and to correct homeostatic disturbances; underlying UTI may have tipped the balance.

INDWELLING CATHETERS AND UTI

Long-term indwelling urinary catheters are used occasionally to control urinary incontinence where other forms of treatment have failed or in some men with prostatic obstruction in whom surgery is contra-indicated. The urinary catheter is known to be the chief source of nosocomial infection of the urinary tract and may lead to bacteriuria, pyelonephritis, bacteraemia and death. Under optimal care the risk of acquiring infection is about 5 to 6 per cent per day and the rate of acquisition for such infection rises in the elderly and sicker subjects. The irritant effect of the catheter head on the bladder mucosa may also breach its defences and form a port of entry for infection. Certainly there is a close relationship between bacteraemia and the presence of indwelling urinary catheters. A closed drainage system may be maintained with sterile urine for a week, or exceptionally for a few days longer than this, but thereafter infection is inevitable. One port of entry is in the connection between the collecting system and the catheter and this should be protected from outside contamination as much as possible. Infections acquired in hospital tend to be due to resistant and uncommon strains of bacteria and maybe by more than one organism. Not only may they provide a hazard to the patient but also to staff handling the catheter and collecting equipment and they add to the endemic bacterial flora in the ward.

Treatment of such infections in the continuing presence of a catheter is inevitably followed by recurrence with the same or a different organism and as long as there are no symptoms of infection no treatment should be given. There is no justification, therefore, for regular laboratory testing of the urine in patients with long-term indwelling urinary catheters. Nor is there any place for prophylactic antimicrobial therapy. Medical treatment should be on a short-term basis if pyelonephritis, bacteraemia or a symptomatic acute episode occurs.

The use of bladder washouts is controversial. They will not diminish the presence of infection even if an antiseptic solution is used. However, they may diminish debris formation and catheter blockage and the substances to be recommended for this purpose are Uro-Tainer Suby-G or Uro-Tainer Solution R (Vifor SA, Geneva, Switzerland/CliniMed Ltd., High Wycombe, Bucks., UK) prepacked washout solutions. One school of thought believes that the use of bladder washouts, by passively distending the bladder after a period during which it has been contracted, may predispose to the entry of organisms through the mucosa. There is however no evidence to support this contention.

PRACTICAL POINTS

● Between 20 and 30 per cent of elderly women and 15 per cent of elderly men have significant bacteriuria.

- The classical presentation of symptoms of UTI in the elderly is the same as in the younger population. However, symptoms are often atypical in old age. Mental confusion is extremely common as are increasing immobility and frequent falls. Classical symptoms may have other causes than infection. Urine cultures are therefore commonly required.

- Faecal incontinence and poor perineal hygiene may be associated factors in the development of urinary tract infection as may outflow obstruction in elderly men. In addition immunological vigour declines with age.

- Catheters may be needed to obtain specimens from some elderly patients especially incontinent or confused women.

- In general a single short-term course of therapy should be given to all patients in whom bacteriuria is encountered for the first time. If symptoms are thereby relieved, further treatment may be necessary should reinfection or relapse occur. If there is no effect on symptoms or if the patient is asymptomatic no further course of treatment should be given even in the case of reinfection or relapse.

- Aggressive treatment may be needed in patients with an initial infection, infection in the presence of renal insufficiency, infection in the presence of glomerular damage, febrile patients with upper tract infection, patients with suspected gram-negative septicaemia and elderly patients presenting acutely with non-specific symptoms in the presence of significant bacteriuria.

- Management should include increased fluid intake and antibiotic therapy. Short courses are acceptable and even desirable in old people.

- Patients who should be referred include ill patients who do not respond to conventional simple measures, patients with suspected septicaemia or peritonitis, patients with complicated UTI and symptomatic patients with infection due to unusual organisms.

● The long-term effect of bacteriuria in the elderly is controversial and remains unresolved.

● Treatment of infections in the continuing presence of a catheter is inevitably followed by recurrence and as long as there are no symptoms no treatment should be given. The use of bladder washouts is controversial. They may diminish debris formation.

References

1. Kunin, C. M. (1979). Guide to examination of the urine. In *Detection, Prevention and Management of Urinary Tract Infections*. 3rd Edition, pp. 57–90. (Philadelphia: Lea and Febiger)
2. Gleckman, R. A. (1982). Urinary tract infection in adults: selective clinical microbiological and therapeutic considerations. In Easmon, C. S. F. and Jeljaszewicz, J. (eds.) *Medical Microbiology 1*. pp. 267–326. (London: Academic Press)
3. Dontas, A. J. (1984). Urinary tract infections and their implications. In Brocklehurst, J. C. (ed.) *Urology in the Elderly*. pp. 162–192. (Edinburgh: Churchill Livingstone)

Further reading

Kass, E. H. and Brumfitt, W. (eds.) (1975). Infections of the urinary tract, *Proceedings of the Third International Symposium on Pyelonephritis*, Royal College of Physicians, London, July 21–23. *Studies in Infectious Disease Research* (Chicago and London: The University of Chicago Press)

Choudhury, S. L. and Brocklehurst, J. C. (1986). Urinary tract infection in old age. In Macias, J. F. and Cameron, J. S. (eds.) *The Kidney in Old Age*. pp. 254–281. (London: Butterworths)

INDEX